SEX AND CONSEQUENCES

*A Bioethical Guide for
Youth and Parents and Teachers*

EDWARD O. SHAKESPEARE

Bloomington, IN 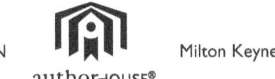 Milton Keynes, UK

authorHOUSE®

AuthorHouse™
1663 Liberty Drive, Suite 200
Bloomington, IN 47403
www.authorhouse.com
Phone: 1-800-839-8640

AuthorHouse™ UK Ltd.
500 Avebury Boulevard
Central Milton Keynes, MK9 2BE
www.authorhouse.co.uk
Phone: 08001974150

First published by AuthorHouse 4/25/2007

ISBN: 978-1-4259-8465-6 (e)
ISBN: 978-1-4259-8464-9 (sc)
ISBN: 978-1-4259-8463-2 (hc)

Library of Congress Control Number: 2006910774

Printed in the United States of America
Bloomington, Indiana

This book is printed on acid-free paper.

Introduction

Did you ever play the childhood game "Truth or Consequences"? It involves having to reveal secrets (like giving the password for admission to one's clubhouse or telling one's true feelings about someone else). If you refused to tell the truth, you suffered unpleasant consequences. If you told the truth, there was no penalty. You discovered, however, that telling the truth had its own consequences (ranging from embarrassment to relief or from anger to joy), depending on how much you pried into each other's lives and feelings. Sometimes you might have thought the game should be called "Truth *and* Consequences."

Who and what we *are*, everything we *do*, and much of what we *think*, have *consequences*. Even when we make decisions and do things alone, sure no one will ever know, we are creating tiny ripples of indirect consequences that affect our character and our moral development (positively or negatively) and eventually affect other people. Becoming *aware* of consequences is a part of growing up.

This book is called ***Sex and Consequences*** because our sexual nature has consequences and, like our curiosity about truth, can evoke joy, embarrassment, anger, relief, tears, laughter, despair, hope. And all these emotional responses are profoundly associated with that most necessary of human emotions, *love*.

Many falsehoods have been written and spoken about sex in human beings, either through ignorance or to defend or condemn certain attitudes and behavior. This book is as truthful as I can make it, and I believe I have successfully avoided superstitions and unreasonable fears and strictures about the subject. Certainly I have availed myself of up-to-date scientific information; and I hope, and think, I have been truthful and objective about the responsibilities and consequences of our sexual nature and behavior. But I have not avoided controversial areas of opinion and judgment. Making moral and ethical decisions that are sensitive to person, to family, and to society (and to the traditions, cultures, and institutions of society) is not always easy, especially when these decisions involve conflicting responsibilities and conflicting consequences.

THE PURPOSES OF THE BOOK

In this book I intend to explain sex, sexuality, and sexual behavior so that you, from pre-teens into adulthood, will become aware of the *personal and social consequences of human sexuality and sexual behavior.* In so doing I hope I am giving you and your parents and your teachers and counselors a helpful basis for discussion and guidance in a vital function of your lives, to help make this part of your lives wonderful and exciting. At the same time, *help you to be caring of others and of yourselves, so that you will be morally responsible and physically and emotionally healthy members of the human family.*

BEFORE WE BEGIN: A SENSITIVITY TO LANGUAGE

One of the difficulties in discussing matters related to sex is that our feelings about the subject are a powerful mix of curiosity and embarrassment. From earliest childhood, for instance, we learn to keep certain parts of our bodies clothed and private. From earliest childhood we also learn that mysterious, vague feelings of pleasure sometimes radiate from these parts of our bodies. This privacy and mystery, and all the conflicting emotions, create problems in vocabulary and factual information. Since we need an adequate vocabulary and factual information to proceed with reasonable, practical, ethical, and moral discussions about sex and sexuality, let's deal first with the problem of vocabulary.

Euphemisms. Words and phrases substituted for blunt reality to protect us from embarrassment or discomfort are called euphemisms. For instance, people may refer euphemistically to the organs of sexual reproduction as "privates" or "private parts." The word "gender," which is a grammatical term for masculine, feminine, and neuter nouns and modifiers in some foreign languages, has become a popular, almost standard, euphemism for the sex of a human being. These euphemisms imply a sensitivity to people's feelings, which is important to getting along with our fellow human beings. Sometimes, however, euphemisms sound foolish or unduly prudish. People who stress mannerly speech might praise your courtesy in using euphemisms, but informal friends who are accustomed to blunt speech might ridicule you. Knowing when and where to use euphemisms and when and where to use more straightforward language is all in the process of acquiring socially responsible maturity. In dealing with sex, sexuality, and sexual behavior in this book, I shall refer to euphemisms only when they need explanation; they are simply not otherwise informative.

Slang. Nor shall I use slang, except when it needs explanation. Since sexual slang may imply violence and disrespect for women and for men, and because it can be misleading or ignorant, it can be grossly offensive. Insensitive, indiscriminate use of sexual slang can produce severe social consequences, even though nowadays it is heard and used with frequency and casualness.

Scientific Vocabulary. Instead, I shall use the informative vocabulary of science, and I shall try to be clear in my use of that vocabulary so that you can be clear in your use of it.

Jokes and Consequences. One other comment about the language of sex. The invention of words and phrases to hide or distort or poke fun at the mysterious, the private, the forbidden gives us opportunities for an endless supply of jokes about sex. Jokes about sex that are clever, humorous, and not disrespectful of people's feelings, can---if indulged in *sparingly* and among accepting people---delight the listener. But jokes that "put down" males or females or use crude language and gross descriptions can embarrass and anger the listener. Such a response indicates that the jokester needs to develop a more sensitive attitude toward listeners. Though intentions may be harmless, the consequences of misjudging your company and what is acceptable in risque jokes can be embarrassing and isolating.

Contents

PART I

Sexually Coming Of Age,
And Its Consequences

THE BIOLOGY OF
SEXUAL REPRODUCTION

Before you get to the information you'll be most directly interested in, you should know something of what science has taught us about reproduction as the basis of life itself. This won't be easy reading, but it is essential to understanding what it is in your *nature* that makes sex so vital and so interesting.

DNA. The most basic characteristic of living things (or living entities) is their ability to *reproduce* themselves. All life on our planet is here because of this essential ability. The earliest life forms, almost four billion years ago, had as their primary building blocks *self-replicating, organic* (organic, meaning they contain the element carbon) *molecules* of so-called **DNA**. DNA, or **d**eoxyribo**n**ucleic **a**cid, the "thread of life," is a complex molecule structured as a **double helix**. This "double helix" is so called because in X-ray diffraction photographs it looks like a ladder twisted around and around itself. Picture the DNA molecule this way (see also Figure 1): The "rails" are strings of energy-producing sugars and phosphates (about which you can learn from biology texts). The "rungs," between the "rails," are couplings of so-called *nucleotides* (shown and named in Figure 1). No one knows how these chemicals, billions of years ago, chanced to cluster in such a way as to make up DNA, but once they did, the DNA began "like mad" to do what comes naturally to DNA---replicate itself. One might say that all the simplest and most complex forms of life, past and present, are evolved from the varied ways in which DNA protects and perpetuates itself.

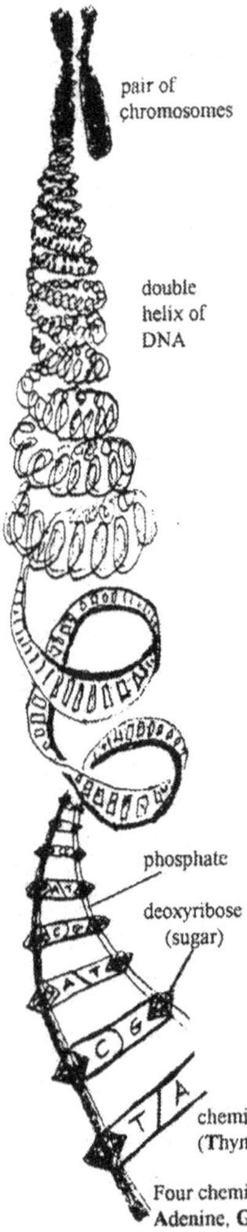

Genes. The mechanisms in DNA that enable reproduced life forms to resemble their parents are the very complicated chemical and physical actions of **genetic material** that is replicated and passed on from generation to generation. This genetic material is in the form of **genes** (arranged as such in the DNA of cells more complicated than bacteria). Genes are special groups of coupled nucleotides (the "rungs" on the DNA "ladder"). They are identifiable parts of self-replicating DNA. Genes are responsible for the way living things develop inheritable characteristics (like color of hair, eyes, and skin, and many, many other characteristics) to pass on from generation to generation. The specific numbers, identities, and placements of genes in the DNA of cells in a living entity are the **genome** of that life form.

Most plant and animal life visible to our eyes reproduces sexually (involving what we call the sexes, male and female). Some smaller life forms---single-cell forms such as bacteria and amoebas---reproduce **asexually**, without sex. But sexual reproduction, as I shall explain, accounts for the amazing variations and differences we see among human individuals and among individuals of other species that reproduce sexually.

pair of chromosomes

double helix of DNA

phosphate

deoxyribose (sugar)

chemical bases (Thymine, Adenine)

Four chemical bases, Thymine, Adenine, Guanine, and Cytosine, provide the grouped combinations that create genes. Thymine always combines with Adenine, Guanine always with Cytosine.

Figure 1. Diagram of DNA

For replication, DNA unzips where the bases are joined. Then each half takes on new bases, phosphates, and sugars.

4

The following explanation is on the molecular science of reproduction. But hold tight: though it's dense reading, you'll find it a rewarding journey into the unfolding mysteries of life itself.

EXPLAINING THE MOLECULAR BASIS OF SEXUAL REPRODUCTION

The many life forms---plant and animal---that reproduce sexually have body parts or separate life forms that we call male and female and which produce special cells called male sex cells and female sex cells. It is these sex cells that get together to produce offspring. The male sex cells are called **sperms**, and the female sex cells are called **eggs**, and this is true of plants as well as animals. A more technical name for an animal sperm is **spermatozoon** (pronounced SPERMatoZOEon), and the plural is spermatozoa. The more technical name for an egg is **ovum** (pronounced OHvum), and the plural is ova.

Now back to DNA, an essential part of every live cell and very much involved in cell division. In each cell of a multicellular life form is a tiny sphere called a **nucleus**. DNA is in the nucleus, and when a cell in a growing life form prepares to divide into two cells (asexually), the DNA organizes itself into *pairs* of tiny cigar-shaped packages called **chromosomes**. Each chromosome is a packed double helix of DNA, and the two chromosomes of a pair have, side-by-side, identical alignments of genes.

When a cell has grown big enough to divide, the membrane surrounding the nucleus disintegrates, and the pairs of chromosomes align themselves across an equatorial plane to replicate themselves. These replicated pairs then pull away from each other into their newly formed cells, where they reside in new nuclei. This kind of cell division is called **mitosis**. The diagrammatic illustration (Figure 2) may help you to see this, but remember that the self-replicating nature of DNA is the driving force behind this cellular activity. (By the way, if you wonder where the ingredients for replication come from, just think of the food you eat, how it's transformed into the molecules that nourish your own cells.)

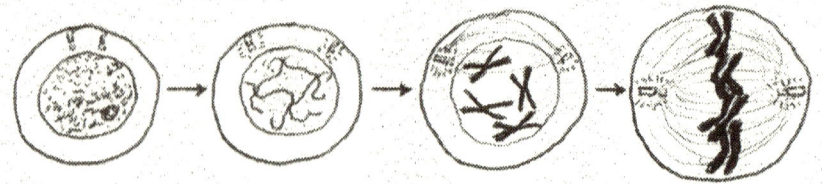

Above: Preparatory to cell division, the chromosomes become less distinct, then elongate into threads. "Polar bodies," outside the nucleus, move toward "poles" of the cell. The chromosomes double, shorten, and thicken. The DNA has replicated itself, and the chromosomes move toward an "equatorial plane."

Below: Aligned at the equatorial plane, the replicated chromosomes pull away from their duplicates. Drawn apart by the polar bodies, they form new nuclei, and the cell completes division.

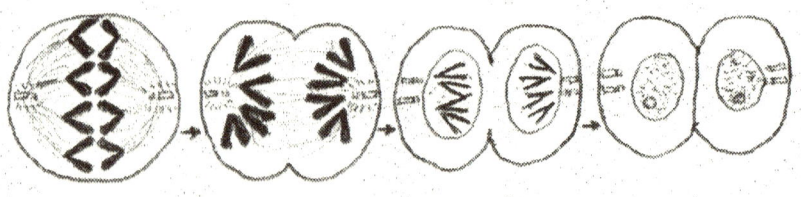

Figure 2. Mitosis. Simplified to show replication
of only four pairs of chromosomes.

In human cells there are 23 pairs of chromosomes. The two chromosomes of each pair, though identical in alignment of genes, are not, however, identical in the DNA of those genes. This is because the DNA of one chromosome of a pair originated in the person's mother, and the DNA of the other chromosome originated in the person's father.

This gets us to *sex* cells. All the cells divide by mitosis except *sex cells*, which divide differently *when they are ready to become sperms in males and eggs in females.* Sperms develop in the testicles, eggs in the ovaries, primary sex organs in males and females.

Now to go on with DNA, chromosomes, and cell division, I ask this question: If there are 23 pairs of chromosomes in each cell in one human generation, why aren't there 46 pairs in the next generation, 92 in the next, and so on? The answer leads us to the source of wonderful variety in all living things that reproduce sexually.

When your body begins to produce eggs or sperms---at puberty and adolescence---these sex cells undergo a special kind of division, called **reduction division** (or **meiosis**). The paired chromosomes clump together as they replicate and pull apart, and in so doing they tangle and cross over, and bits and pieces of the paired chromosomes, from your mother and father, get transferred from one replicating chromosome of a pair to the other of the pair. Moreover, when the final division occurs, the newly constituted chromosome pairs pull *apart* and go *separately* into each newly-formed mature sex cell. Thus a mature sex cell contains *only half the number of chromosomes*---no longer a pair. The diagrammatic illustration (Figure 3) may help to explain meiosis. The importance of the "half number of chromosomes" will help to answer the question in the paragraph above, as you will later see. But first, a further significance of reduction division.

Reduction division is the ultimate sexual union. This is when your mother and father get together on a *molecular* level, long after the loving sexual intercourse that produced you. And all the time you are producing eggs or sperms, your parents' DNA (and their parents' DNA) is getting spliced into new combinations. Hence the variety in life forms that reproduce sexually. Thus every individual differs from all other individuals and even brothers or sisters in the same family look and act differently.

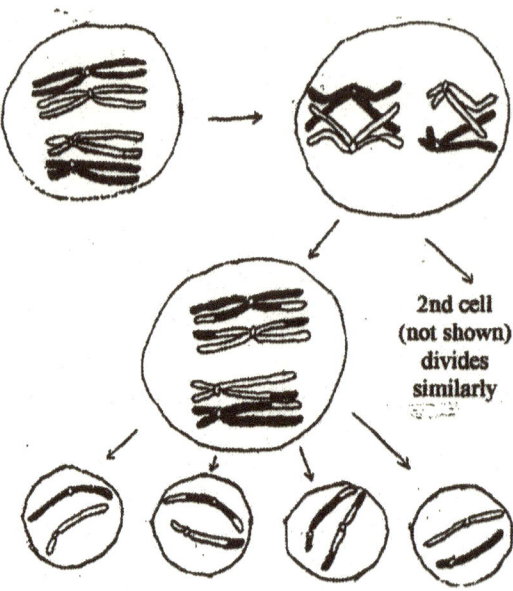

Figure 3. Meiosis. **Top left:** Immature sex cell contains 2 pairs of chromosomes (black) from one parent, 2 pairs (white) from other parent. **Top right:** Chromosomes tangle along equatorial plane; cell ready to divide. **Center:** Chromosomes of 2 resulting cells (only one shown) have mixed parental parts. **Bottom:** Reduction division produces 4 mature sex cells, each containing half the chromosome pairs.

Now I have to back up a little. Remember that in human beings every living cell (except mature sex cells) has 23 *pairs* of chromosomes. Each pair has genes that determine the development of different structures and characteristics of a person. One of the 23 pairs has genes that are the sex determiner. Under an electron microscope the two chromosomes of the sex-determining pair in a *female* look identical. Biologists name them the **XX pair**. In a *male*, however, the two chromosomes of the sex-determining pair are *not* look-alikes. One looks identical to an X chromosome (in fact, it *is* an X chromosome), but the other is a runt. The runt lacks many of the genes in the X. This smaller chromosome of the sex-determining pair in the male is called a **Y chromosome**, and the pair is called the **XY pair**. In a human female every living cell (except mature eggs) has an XX pair of chromosomes. In a human male every living cell (except mature sperms) has an XY pair of chromosomes.

When a human female matures into adolescence and some of her egg cells begin to mature, undergoing *reduction division*, a mature egg cell, or ovum (with only half of each pair of chromosomes) will have only one X chromosome. But when a human male matures into adolescence and his sperm cells begin to mature, undergoing *reduction division*, a mature spermatozoon, with only half of each pair of chromosomes, will have *either* an X chromosome *or* a Y chromosome. So in females all mature ova will have the X chromosome, but in males 50 percent of mature spermatozoa will have the X chromosome, and 50 percent will have the Y chromosome.

Finally we get to answer the question about keeping human chromosome pairs at 23. When a mature spermatozoon, with only half of each pair, fertilizes a mature ovum, with only half of each pair, the chromosome count is restored to 23 pairs, and there's a fifty-fifty chance of producing an XX girl or an XY boy.

I've gone into all this detail because the science of genetics is more and more in the news, especially news about human chromosomes and the **genome**, so you really ought to be acquainted with this knowledge. All this is shown in two excellent videos, *Cracking the Code of Life* and *Life's Greatest Miracle* (see Bibliography).

SEXUAL ATTRACTION

How do the male and female sex cells find each other? Biology text books provide fascinating examples of remarkable conditions under which male sex cells of an organism find their way to the female sex cells produced by another organism (sometimes another part of the same organism, as in flowers) of the same species. Chance and coincidence play a significant role (think of pollination by wind, for instance). And so does the remarkable evolutionary interdependence of organisms within a particular environment. Consider, as an example, how some flowering plants are dependent on insects for pollination.

In many sexually reproducing organisms, both plant and animal, sex cells from the male are produced in superabundance, and chance---rather than mating as *we* think of it---brings male sex cells close enough to female sex cells for uniting.

Among mammals that have a "mating season," or a time of "heat," the female produces mature eggs only at that time. During heat she gives off odors (not consciously controlled) that are strongly attractive to the male of the species. The male is so attracted that he mates with the female, discharging his sperms into her receiving organ. The sperms from the male have thus a short internal distance to travel toward the egg, or eggs, of the female. Vital to the *final* uniting of sperm and egg from male and female parents is the egg's attraction of the sperm. The surface of the egg emits chemicals that spread out and are attractive to spermatozoa, and sperms have built-in biochemical locaters for that attraction.

Human Sexual Attraction

Human sexual attraction is not regulated by a mating season or a time of heat. It develops instead from *discovery*, *curiosity*, and *learning*. Infants *discover*, for instance, that to touch and fondle the external sex organs produces a pleasant feeling.

By the way, another name for sex organs is **genitals** (pronounced JENituls) or **genitalia** (jeniTAILeeuh). I shall use these terms interchangeably.

Parents discourage their children from fondling their external genitals and also insist that genitals---more than any other parts of the body---be covered with clothing. Thus children *learn* that there is something special about their genitals, something associated with pleasure but also with privacy and modesty. Of course, these responses arouse *curiosity*. Boys and girls, even when they are very little, are curious not only about their own genitals but also about the differences between male and female genitals.

Boys and girls also *learn* that disrespectful and rudely aggressive attempts to satisfy sexual curiosity can be embarrassing, even frightening.

Parents worry about such incidents, and that is why they may discourage their children from sex play. Feelings of guilt, therefore, are associated with the feelings of pleasure and adventure in the discoveries of sexual attraction. These are some of the *vital consequences* associated with human sexual behavior: We would not reproduce if there were no pleasure and adventure in sexual attraction, but our upbringing and our intelligence should give us the sensitivity as social human beings to enjoy that attraction within respectful bounds.

Most of human sexual behavior, including the early discovery and curiosity stages, is *learned.* It is learned from parents and other family members. It is learned from friends. It is learned from courses and discussions taught in schools, churches, synagogues, and other respected institutions. It is learned from books. It is learned from observation, seeing the mating behavior of cats, dogs, and farm animals. And, unfortunately, it is learned from exposure to pornography and similar sources that make huge profits through arousing crude and insensitive desires. In fact, the ready accessibility of pornography on the Internet is a clear and present danger to the healthy and happy sexual development of young people.

What we learn and how we learn it have their consequences. I shall say more about that as you read further in this book.

THE BIOLOGY OF SEXUAL
DEVELOPMENT IN THE HUMAN BEING

In order to learn more about human sexual reproduction, you must first know more about the human male and the human female.

THE HUMAN FEMALE

The Anatomy of the Sex Organs. The sex of the female infant is immediately distinguishable from that of the male infant. In the area of the groin are two swellings of flesh pressed gently against each other These two swellings are called **lips**. If the lips are parted, they reveal a **vestibule** that has two openings---toward the front a tiny opening for urination, and behind it a larger opening for sexual functions. The lips and the vestibule are called the **vulva** (the first syllable rhyming with *wool*) or the *external genitalia of the female* (see Figure 4).

The larger of the two openings in the vestibule is the entrance to an elastic passageway called the **vagina** (vaJYnuh). Beginning here, the genitals are referred to as the *internal genitalia* (see Figures 4 and 5). At the inner end of the vagina is the **womb** (woom) or **uterus** (YOOterus). The uterus is shaped like an upside-down pear. Its smaller, lower end bulges slightly into the inner end of the vagina. This bulge is called the **cervix** (SIRvix). The tip of the cervix has an opening into the interior of the uterus. The uterus, normally no larger than a small pear, is the organ that holds the developing baby-to-be and can expand considerably. On either side of the upper, wider end of the uterus is a narrow tube called the **fallopian tube**, or **oviduct**. Each oviduct flares out at its far end into a fringed hood that appears to embrace an oval organ called an **ovary** (Ovuree). In an infant each ovary is approximately the size of an irregularly shaped grape; in a mature woman it's the size of an irregularly shaped, large ripe olive. The two ovaries are the primary female *reproductive* organs, also known as the female **gonads** (GOnads). They produce the tiny female sex cells (eggs, or ova) that, if fertilized by the male sex cells (sperms), will initiate the process toward the production of a new human being. All these organs are the **primary sex characteristics** of the human female.

Now the vulva is more complicated than I first explained (see Figure 6). The fleshy swellings, or lips, are **outer** or **major lips** (*labia majora* in Latin). On their inner side, immediately surrounding the urinary opening and the vagina, is a thinner pair of lips, called **inner** or **minor lips** (*labia minora* in Latin). The inner lips join at the front end of the vestibule (forward of the urinary opening) to form a small hood. This hood, or **foreskin**, covers, or partially covers, a small, bud-like organ, the **clitoris** (CLIToris). The clitoris is richly supplied with nerve endings and small blood vessels, and it is the focus for the pleasurable sensations essential to sexual attraction.

One other structure of the vulva is the **hymen** (HIGHmen), a thin membrane that partially covers the entrance to the vagina. This membrane, also known as the *maidenhead* or, in slang, *cherry*, may not last beyond childhood, especially if a girl is strenuously athletic; but since it is the subject of folklore and misinformation about sexual behavior, I shall say more about it later.

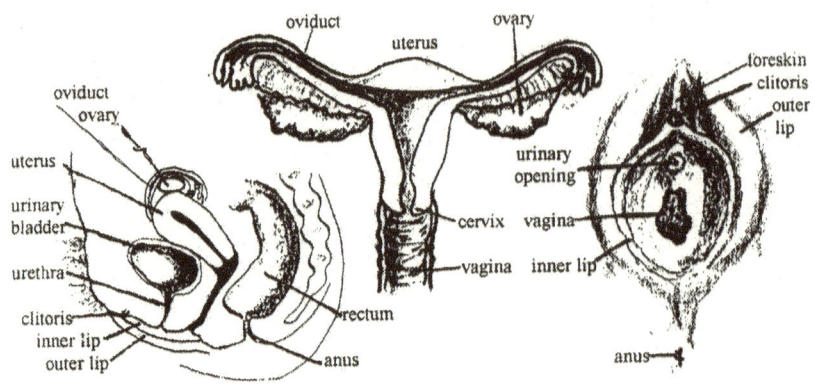

Figure 5. Left: Female reproductive organs, side view, internal.
Figure 4. Center: Female reproductive organs, front view, internal.
Figure 6. Right: The vulva and vestibule, with lips parted.

PUBERTY AND ADOLESCENCE IN THE HUMAN FEMALE

The Physiology of the Sex Organs

The female reproductive organs do not function as such until **puberty** (PYOObertee). *Puberty* is the time during which sex organs develop toward fully functioning organs of reproduction. Its time span is about three to four years, and in girls it begins usually between the ages of 11 and 16, when certain internal glands begin to secrete greatly increased quantities of special biochemicals directly into the bloodstream. These glands are called **endocrine** (ENdoekrin) **glands**. Their secretions are called **hormones**.

The endocrine gland that starts the process of puberty is the **hypothalamus** (hypoTHALamus), a small part of the brain above the **pituitary gland**. Hormones from the hypothalamus cause the pituitary gland to produce hormones which stimulate the ovaries to grow and to produce **estrogen** (EStrojen). Estrogen hormones are most directly associated with the onset of puberty. (Note that ovaries function as endocrine glands in addition to producing ova.) Another endocrine gland, the adrenal (adREENul), lying on each kidney, secretes in girls as well as boys a small quantity of **androgen** (ANdrojen) hormones, which also stimulate the process of puberty. When the "biological clock" in the hypothalamus triggers these endocrine glands, a girl begins her journey into womanhood.

The beginning of puberty, stimulated by estrogens from the ovaries (and the much smaller amount of androgens from the adrenal glands) is noticeable first in a tenderness of breast tissue in the area of the nipples, followed by gradual increase in breast size. This may begin as early as age 10 or as late as age 15, but usually around 11 or 12. Then the vulva begins to enlarge: the outer and inner lips, the clitoris, and the vaginal opening. Meanwhile, the external area just in front of the vulva increases in fleshiness. This is called the **mons veneris** (literally the "Mount of Venus"). Downy hair then appears on the mons veneris and on the outer sides of the outer lips. This hair is called **pubic hair**.

All these changes are called the development of **secondary sex characteristics**. They appear so gradually that a girl may not be aware at first of what is happening.

Menarche. The most *significant event* of puberty occurs approximately two years after the first tenderness in the nipple area. It is an event for which every girl should be prepared. It is distinguished by a small but significant flow of blood from the vagina: **menarche** (meNARkee), the first **menstruation**. Menarche is a girl's passage to womanhood---an event to be proud of, an event that a mother may want to celebrate with her daughter.

Menstruation is so much a part of the reproductive years of womanhood that boys and girls and men and women deserve a full explanation, and here it is.

Menstruation and Its Significance. Menstruation occurs approximately every four weeks. It is essential to the reproductive process. When a girl becomes *pubescent*, (begins the years of puberty), the pituitary hormones, triggered by the hypothalamus, stimulate the ovaries to grow (eventually to about the size of a slightly flattened, large ripe olive) and to secrete their own hormones, **estrogen** and, *periodically*, another hormone, **progesterone** (proJESterone), which is directly associated with menstruation.

Now, I'm going to tell you more than you may be interested to know. I include this information because you should be clearly informed how endocrine glands are dependent upon each other in a remarkably complex way. What affects one endocrine gland is likely to affect others, sometimes in unpredictable ways. Therefore, injections or pills involving hormones should be prescribed with great care. Illegal use of hormones puts one at great risk. So read the small indented type to see the interaction of hormones on menstruation.

First, the pituitary hormone **FSH** (follicle stimulating hormone) stimulates the growth of the ovaries and the development of the egg cells and the cells that surround the egg cells within the ovary. The ovaries then secrete **estrogens**, and these estrogens cause growth of nipple tissue, growth of external genitalia, growth of the uterus (to the size of a small pear (about 3 inches long), and increased rate of general body growth. As the ovaries mature to adult size and function, the menstrual cycle begins. Each month (approximately) one immature ovum (egg) divides by reduction division to produce one ripe ovum with a nucleus in which *the paired chromosomes are halved*, and the ovarian cells surrounding this ripening egg form a capsule called a **follicle.**

At this point, the ovaries secrete more and more estrogens into the bloodstream. Eventually the estrogen-in-blood level is high enough to cause a reaction in the pituitary gland. The pituitary gland reduces its secretion of FSH and begins to secrete **LH** (luteinizing hormone). Luteinizing hormone stimulates the ovarian follicle to secrete the hormone **progesterone**. (During this process the cells of the follicle acquire a yellowish color and are called the **corpus luteum**, Latin for *yellow body*. Hence the name *luteinizing* hormone.)

In a fully functioning, female reproductive system this sequence of hormonal secretions and reactions causes the discharge of a ripe ovum from the ripest follicle in one or the other ovary, a process called **ovulation**. The discharged ovum enters the oviduct and begins its descent into the uterus. Menstruation follows ovulation by about 14 days---*if the ovum is not fertilized*.

Menstruation is annoying and often embarrassing for women, but here is why it is essential to the reproductive process.

As I stated in the small print, the pituitary hormone FSH (follicle stimulating hormone) stimulates the ovaries to produce estrogens so that one or the other ovary will produce a single mature ovum from among the thousands of immature ova in the ovaries. Meanwhile, estrogens cause the inner lining of the uterus, the **endometrium** (endoMEEtreeum), to thicken and become rich with tiny blood vessels. The endometrium of the uterus is thus being prepared to receive and nourish an embryo in case that egg has been fertilized by a male sex cell (spermatozoon).

The process of expulsion of a mature ovum from an ovary is called **ovulation** (AHvyooLAYshun), as I stated in the small print above. It is usually a painless event, but it is sometimes accompanied by some pain in the lower abdomen. This pain is called **mittelschmerz** (MITelshmerts), a German word meaning *midpain.*

Ovulation is triggered by the pituitary hormone LH (luteinizing hormone). After ovulation, LH stimulates the now empty ovarian follicle to secrete the hormone **progesterone**. Progesterone stimulates the endometrium to become even richer in blood vessels and in nutritious secretions.

Approximately fourteen days after ovulation the ovaries stop secreting estrogen and progesterone *if the expelled egg has not been fertilized,*. This causes the newly-formed blood vessels and nutritious cells in the thickened endometrium to die. The dead material, including the unfertilized ovum, then sloughs away from the rest of the endometrium and, with some bleeding, washes out of the uterus, down through the vagina, to the vulva and outside. This sloughing and bleeding is called **menstruation** or, because it occurs periodically, the **period**.

The Menstrual Cycle. Time lapse from menstruation to menstruation is about 28 days. This is called the menstrual cycle. Ovulation occurs at midcycle, on or about the fourteenth day after the *beginning* of menstruation.

How Pregnancy Interrupts the Cycle. If a sperm fertilizes the ovum, usually within the 24 hours after ovulation, the fertilized ovum will begin to develop into a tiny multicellular sphere, the **blastula** stage of an **embryo**, as it descends down the oviduct and into the uterus. By the time it enters the uterus, this embryo will have an outer layer of cells that enable it to invade the thickened, nutritious endometrium. Thus this tiny cluster of cells actually burrows into the uterine wall and develops there. At this point, about 10 days after fertilization, its outermost cells secrete *their own hormones*, which enter the uterine bloodstream. These hormones stimulate the ovaries to *continue* secreting estrogen and progesterone. Thus menstruation ceases while the cell cluster develops into an **embryo** in the uterus, and the uterus remains a nutritious environment. If all goes well, this time of development---from fertilized egg to embryo to **fetus** (FEEtus) to birth of an **infant**---lasts 9 months and is called **gestation** (jesTAYshun), and the mother during this time is said to be **pregnant**.

Coping with Menstruation. Though a process of nature, menstruation is unpleasant and inconvenient. It occurs, on average, every 28 days, interrupted only by pregnancy or by unusual emotional or physical stress, until it ceases entirely (**menopause**) in a woman's late 40s or early 50s. But every woman knows that the menstrual cycle does not proceed with clockwork regularity. It is irregular during the first year or so after menarche, and even after that it may fluctuate from longer to shorter cycles. Moreover, the menstrual flow may differ from cycle to cycle, sometimes heavy, sometimes scant; sometimes lasting only 3 days, sometimes a week. And menstruation may be accompanied by painful "cramps" in the lower abdominal, or pelvic, region.

In some girls and women another source of discomfort is **premenstrual syndrome (PMS)**, inexplicable feelings of nervousness, anger, depression, and fatigue, sometimes accompanied by headache and puffiness, coming on a few hours or days before menstruation. Adolescents and adult women who suffer from PMS should list their symptoms and seek medical advice for relief.

Girls should be well informed about menstruation before menarche occurs. Thoughtful parents, school counselors, and the family medical adviser can prevent the fear and embarrassment that ignorance, superstition, and misinformation can provoke.

Also vital is proper instruction in the use of absorbent pads during menstruation. Some pads are worn externally, fitting over the vulva. Others are cylindrical, for insertion in the vagina. Choice will depend on athletic activities and on personal comfort, but medical advice should be sought too, for sanitary precautions are very important. Another consideration in being prepared for menstruation is to know how and where to dispose of used pads. Written instructions that come with the pads are helpful, and so---especially---are parents and counselors.

Girls should rehearse with parents and counselors how to deal with circumstances affecting their privacy and dignity during menstruation. For instance, girls should inform athletics coaches at times of menstruation, and they may want to back off from discomforting swimming or social activities. A girl may be briefly informative, saying she is having her period or suffering cramps; or she may be more euphemistic, saying simply she doesn't feel up to doing whatever is called for.

Adults and peers should respect the privacy and dignity of a girl or woman who is menstruating. Boys and men bear a special responsibility to be respectful, since they do not share in this biological phenomenon. It is an insensitive boy or man who makes menstruation the subject of gossip and sniggers.

Completion of Puberty in the Female

During the next two years, while the **primary sex characteristics** are maturing, the **secondary sex characteristics** continue developing. The voice becomes richer and slightly deeper. Pubic hair becomes coarse and curly, growing also in the area surrounding the anus. Hair begins to grow in the armpits (**axillary hair**) and on the legs. (In many cultures women shave axillary hair and leg hair; and if they wear thongs and skimpy swimming clothes, they remove pubic hair that might show.) Meanwhile, a great increase in general body growth occurs. Hips widen and breasts and body begin to acquire a woman's shape in the full development of primary and secondary sex characteristics.

PSYCHOLOGICAL IMPLICATIONS OF ADOLESCENCE IN GIRLS

Now I must say more about puberty and menstruation, and I must define adolescence. **Adolescence** begins with puberty and ends several years after puberty is completed. Adolescence is said to be completed when a person has acquired not only sexual maturity but also a sense of mature self-identity and the ability to mingle and compete comfortably with adults. That may be as early as age 18 in some people and as late as 24 in others.

Differences in Maturation. Adolescence is a time of emotional, intellectual, and whole-body change, as well as a time of sexual development. As you have seen, it can begin with puberty as early as age 10 for some girls (even earlier for a few). The average age for *menarche* is between 11 and 13. Girls who enter puberty early grow rapidly taller than their friends and classmates, and they may feel awkward and out of place. They may strike up friendships with older girls who are at about the same stage of pubertal development. This causes ruptures and hurt feelings in old friendships. The pubescent girl feels more mature and thinks differently from her prepubescent friend. The prepubescent friend feels abandoned by a dear friend who has become a stranger. These are stresses that girls must be sensitive to. A word of kindness, a gesture of friendship from the more mature girl can help to relieve the unhappiness. The less mature girl has a responsibility too; she must understand that puberty is a time when such changes occur, and she must be forgiving.

In addition to age differences in the onset of puberty, there are differences in the ways girls grow and develop in puberty. Some girls seem to blossom immediately into beautiful young women. They look like TV and movie ideals. On the surface, and to the casual observer, this may seem to be wonderfully good luck, but it can have its disadvantages, as I shall point out later. Most girls, however, go through a temporary awkward stage, during which they may be taller and more angular than desired, or shorter and fatter, or some other unwished for combination. Temporarily, too, facial features may grow out of proportion, and hormonal influences on complexion may cause acne.

Accepting Differences. Even more distressing is the emotional pain caused by our society's emphasis on slenderness and on breast size and shape. It is difficult enough for girls to compare their mirror images with the standards set by advertisers and the clothing-design industry. Worse is the ridicule girls can inflict on each other, even if it is intended only in jest. Much worse are the crude and insensitive remarks boys may make in attempts to shock girls and show off to their male peers. Parents, teachers, counselors, and especially peers have an obligation to make girls and boys acutely aware of the *consequential* pain of ridicule.

The one constant in female adolescence is that every female differs from every other female, even after reaching full sexual maturity. Some young women are lean and athletic, others more rounded in distribution of body fat. Some have visible downy facial hair and plentiful growth of hair on legs and armpits. Others have only the finest of downy body hair except at the pubis and armpits. Some have large breasts, others small. Some breasts have a large **areola**, the darker, raised area surrounding the nipple; others small. And the areola and nipple may be much darker than the breast or only slightly darker. Even external genitalia differ, in size, shape, and color, especially the inner lips of the vulva. In some women the inner lips are the color of the surrounding flesh, in others slightly or much darker. They may also vary in size and shape, and one lip may be larger than the other. Pubic hair may differ in density, coarseness, and distribution.

Here might be the place to say more about the hymen, so named after Hymen, the Greek god of marriage. It, too, differs in appearance. It may cover most or only a little of the entrance to the vagina. In girls into athletics, it is likely to rupture, causing mild, brief pain and some bleeding---clearly worth reporting to the athletics coach or phys-ed teacher and to parents, but usually inconsequential. In folklore an intact hymen has been considered proof of virginity. There are therefore many jokes about the "maidenhead" or the "cherry" (a slang term that makes no sense), but few girls reach womanhood with hymens still intact, so lack of a hymen is not an indication of "lost virginity."

Human society depends on the sensitive respect of individuals for each other. It also depends on strength of character, a willingness to stand up as an individual and show respect and kindness rather than a yielding attitude of going along with the crowd. Therefore, the maturing girl, developing toward womanhood, should weigh the *consequences of cruelty* against the *consequences of kindness*. My hope, and one of the purposes of this book, is that she will reject temptations to tease and scorn her less developed peers and remember that biological development is mostly beyond control.

Sense of humor and lively interest in studies, hobbies, sports, and organizations of service to other people can do much to overcome miseries of adolescence, and are vital to the development of one's social and intellectual skills. Friends and strangers overlook all sorts of physical awkwardness when personality is outgoing---conscious of, and interested in, other people, and not *self*-conscious. Besides, the sources of embarrassment and worry diminish during the final stages of adolescence.

Sexual Urge and Maturing Intellect. While physical changes of puberty are occurring, sex hormones are also stimulating psychological changes. The pubescent girl feels mysteriously attracted to pubescent boys and girls and may discover they too are attracted to her. She is curious to observe the development of her own body. Her curiosity about sex intensifies. She may become infatuated with a particular boy, or, as happens with some girls, she may feel so attracted to boys in general that her peers may call her "boy crazy." These changes, part of the biological mechanisms that ensure sexual reproduction, are complex and stressful, however, so more about them in Part II.

Intellectual changes also take place. An adolescent girl discovers that her ability to think abstractly about values, morals, and ethics has greatly expanded. The *consequences* of sexual maturity depend on one's thinking about values and morals and ethics.

I shall return to this theme, but first I must say something about the human male and how he develops through puberty and adolescence. *Consequences of sexual maturity and behavior depend on our understanding of both sexes.*

The Human Male

The human male's sex is set by a pair of sex-determining chromosomes called the XY pair (see page 8-9). The Y member of the pair, so-called because it differs from its X counterpart in genetic makeup, is responsible for male sex determination. Every cell in a male's body except mature sperms has the XY pair. Through reduction division mature sperms have only half of each pair, so the X chromosome is in 50 percent of mature sperms and the Y in the other 50 percent.

The Anatomy of the Sex Organs. The features distinguishing the human male are immediately observable at birth. At the groin, or crotch, is a fleshy cylinder, the **penis**, and behind it is a wrinkled sac, the **scrotum** (SKROHtum). At the end of the **shaft** of the penis is a round head, the **glans** (glanz) or **glans penis**. The glans, like the clitoris in the female, is richly supplied with nerve endings and small blood vessels and is a focus for the pleasurable sensations that make sexual reproduction attractive. At the tip of the head is a small vertical mouth, through which urine is passed and through which sperms are discharged when the male's sexual development has enabled him to produce sperms.

Covering all but the tip of the glans is a circular fold of skin, the **foreskin** or **prepuce** (PREEpus). This is surgically removed from the penises of most male infants a few days after birth in an operation called **circumcision** (literally, "cutting around"). On the circumcised penis the glans is fully exposed. Jewish religious ritual requires circumcision, as described in the Torah and in the Old Testament of the Bible. Among people of most other religions, circumcision of males is not required; but failure to keep the inside surface of the foreskin clean can cause discomfort and infection, so most penises are circumcised.

The penis, which is usually limp, can, under certain circumstances, swell and stretch stiffly upward. This is called **erection** and is explained on page 27.

The scrotum contains two ovoid organs called **testicles** or **testes** ((TESteez). These are the primary male *reproductive* organs, also known as male **gonads**. In a baby boy each testicle, or testis, is no larger than a small grape. In a mature male it is the size of a large ripe olive. The interior of a testicle is dense with coils of very narrow tubes called **seminiferous tubules**. At puberty the testicles enlarge and start producing the microscopically small male sex cells, **sperms**, or **spermatozoa**. A mature spermatozoon has a head (containing a nucleus with its halved number of chromosomes) and a tail. The tail enables the sperm to swim in a fluid, **semen** (SEEmen), which I shall describe later.

Those interested in biological detail may want to read the small print below.

> The testicles are suspended in the scrotal sac by **spermatic cords**, which originate in the pelvis. Thus the testicles are outside the body cavity. Through some quirk of evolution, the production of spermatozoa must be at a temperature slightly below body temperature. The scrotum, which has many tiny muscles just under its skin, serves as a temperature regulator. In cold conditions these muscles contract and the scrotal skin wrinkles. At the same time a fine network of musculature (the **cremaster**) on the spermatic cords and enveloping the testicles contracts, and the scrotum tightens against the body. In warm conditions these muscles relax, the skin unwrinkles, and the scrotum hangs lower (allowing a greater surface for cooling by sweat evaporation).

The seminiferous tubules lead from each testicle into a wider coiled tube that forms a soft mass against the exterior of the testicle.

This mass is called the **epididymis** (epeeDIDimis). The epididymis opens into a still wider tube, the **vas deferens**, which enters the pelvic (hip) area inside the body.

The vas deferens and accompanying blood vessels that nourish each testicle and epididymis are ensheathed in tissue to form the spermatic cord (mentioned in small print above), part of which is also the fine network of cremaster musculature (also in the small print above).

Inside the pelvic area the vas deferens makes a U-turn alongside the urinary bladder. Each vas deferens then bends centrally toward a chestnut-shaped gland just below the bladder. This gland is called the **prostate gland**. Close to the prostate gland each vas deferens expands into a pocket-like reservoir, called a

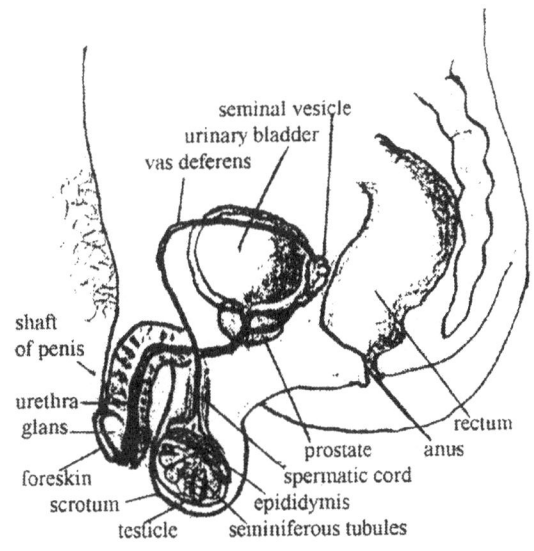

Figure 7. Male reproductive organs, side view.

seminal vesicle. Just beyond the seminal vesicles, the vasa deferentia (plural for vas deferens), are called **ejaculatory** (eeJAKyoolatory) **ducts**. They enter the prostate gland. Inside the prostate gland the ejaculatory ducts join into a single, central tube, the **urethra** (yooREETHra), which passes through the penis to its mouth. (See Figure 7.)

The male's urethra is the tube through which urine passes and also through which spermatozoa, in their special fluid, pass to the outside. (In contrast, the female's urethra is exclusively for passage of urine.) Semen is described in the next section, "Puberty and Adolescence in the Human Male." It is important to know at this point that when a male urinates, he cannot eject semen. Similarly, when he discharges semen, he cannot urinate.

25

The Physiology of the Sex Organs

These **primary sex organs** do not function as such until *puberty*. Puberty in boys begins on average a year later than in girls but spans about the same number of years, 3-4. It is triggered by the **hypothalamus**, a part of the brain that stimulates the **pituitary gland** to secrete the hormones **FSH** and **LH** (see page 16, the small print). In boys FSH stimulates the growth of the testicles and stimulates the seminiferous tubules to produce the sex cells that multiply and ripen into millions of mature spermatozoa. LH also stimulates the testicles to produce **androgens** (hormones that generate masculine looks), principally **testosterone**. Testosterone accelerates the appearance of **secondary sexual characteristics** in males. These characteristics develop as follows. Beginning, on average, at age 12 (in some boys as early as 10 or as late as 17), the testicles begin to enlarge. A year later downy hair appears on the lower abdomen, just above the penis. This coarsens and becomes dense and curly within another year or two. As with the female, it is called **pubic hair**, and it grows also on the scrotum and spreads behind the scrotum and around the anus. During this time the penis grows larger. Then a marked increase in general body growth begins: shoulders broaden, height increases, the chest deepens and widens, and muscular bulk increases. A downy moustache may begin to appear, and **axillary hair** (hair in the armpits) begins to grow.

Anatomy and Physiology of Erection. Erections are spontaneous; they cannot be willed to occur. In infants they are often associated with the need to urinate (as anyone who has bathed a baby boy or changed his diapers knows). They also occur as a regular pattern of sleep in boys, youths, and adults. These kinds of erections are not due to sexual excitement, though the sensation of stiffness may produce sexual excitement. Erections directly related to sexual function are caused by accidental or intentional friction or pressure on the penis and especially by sexually exciting thoughts, dreams, and activities. Since erection gets a great deal of publicity nowadays in print, radio, TV, movies, and especially advertisements by pharmaceutical companies, the following small print is for readers who may want to know more about its anatomy and physiology.

Beneath its skin, the penile shaft is made up mostly of three cylinders, each containing a remarkable arrangement of small arteries and veins and spongy spaces through which blood flows. One cylinder, longer and narrower than the other two, runs the entire center length of the underside of the penis and projects into the glans, or head. Through it runs the urethra. The other two, thicker cylinders, lie side by side above the central one. They too run the length of the shaft but stop short of the head. These three cylinders are called the **corpora cavernosa** (Latin for "cavernous bodies"; the singular is *corpus cavernosum*).

Upon occasion there will be a sudden increase of blood flow into the corpora cavernosa. The spongy cylinders then fill with blood faster than the veins can drain them. This causes **erection**. Erection ceases when the pressure of blood flow into the corpora cavernosa lessens and the veins drain. The penis then returns to its usual limp state.

Even though an erection cannot be willed, the penis becomes erect with little stimulation. This response is called **potency**. Sometimes, however, a boy or man fails to achieve erection when he wishes and expects to, mostly because of nervousness, anxiety, worry, tiredness, or similar distractions. This is usually a temporary condition, but it can create its own anxiety, and when it does, the condition may last longer and be referred to as **impotence** (IMpot'nce) or **erectile dysfunction**. I mention this specifically because many of you have read and seen ads for prescribed drugs in pill form which affect the blood and nervous systems so that males can easily achieve erection. The penis must be stiff in order to penetrate the vagina. The attractiveness of pills that enhance sexual intercourse, and the many jokes about them, make these drugs subject to blackmarketing; but they are powerful drugs that must be prescribed by a licensed doctor, and anyone taking them without prescription runs a serious risk of life-threatening reactions.

The Secretion and Discharge of Semen. By the time pubic hair appears, in addition to growth of penis and testicles, the young male becomes capable of secreting the fluid in which spermatozoa can be discharged from the penis. This fluid is called semen, as I mentioned earlier, or **seminal** (SEMinal) **fluid**. Semen is a yellowish-white, translucent fluid, thick and slippery in consistency.

Of the several organs involved in production of semen, the *seminiferous tubules* secrete a very small quantity to allow spermatozoa to pass into the *epididymis* alongside each testicle. Each epididymis secretes an additional small amount of seminal fluid, enabling spermatozoa to flow through the *vasa deferentia* into the *seminal vesicles*. The seminal vesicles secrete and store much of the bulk of semen. The *prostate gland*, into which the vesicles empty, adds a final, milky, somewhat lesser amount. At the root of the penis, just behind the scrotum, are small glands (*bulbo-urethral glands,* also known as *Cowper's glands*) which, shortly before discharge of semen, secrete into the *urethra* a few drops of clear, colorless, slippery fluid called *pre-ejaculatory fluid.*

At peak sexual excitement, as in sexual intercourse, semen---together with millions of spermatozoa---is secreted and squeezed into the urethra and discharged, **ejaculated** (eeJAKyooLAYted), from the penis. The semen discharged at any one time is technically referred to as the **ejaculate** (eeJAKyulet), and it amounts to approximately a teaspoonful.

Wet Dreams. The pubescent boy's emergence into sexual maturity, nearly two years after the first signs of puberty, will be marked by his first ejaculation. This usually occurs at night, during sleep. The boy may be awakened by a sexually exciting dream ending in an intensely pleasurable pressure in the groin and then several rhythmic spurts of liquid through his erect penis. If he is awakened, he will discover he has discharged a small quantity of slippery, thick fluid, the semen described above. If he sleeps through the event, he will be puzzled to discover in the morning a dried, starchy stain on his sleepwear pants and probably on the bed sheet.

Such an event is called a **nocturnal emission** or **wet dream**. The intense pleasure is called an **orgasm**. A wet dream is involuntary; it cannot be willed, and it cannot be stopped. Nothing to be ashamed of, it should be a source of pride in entering manhood. Parents expect it to occur in their maturing sons, so there is no point in trying to conceal or wash away the stain on bedclothes.

Unlike urine, which accumulates until the bladder must be emptied, semen is secreted mostly during sexual excitement. Except for an occasion of strong sexual excitement, semen does not accumulate to the point at which the male will ejaculate. Wet dreams are usually the consequence of pressure on sleep erections, though a full bladder may be a contributing factor. Urination and ejaculation are distinctly separate from each other, however, so a boy should not fear that his body will confuse the two functions.

Masturbation. In the adolescent male the function of his sex organs and the arousal of his sexual desire are sources of anxiety, curiosity, pride, and pleasure. Just as girls and boys need to know about menstruation and a girl's entrance into womanhood, they should also know about ejaculation and a boy's entrance into manhood.

Since boys have less privacy among each other than girls have, they are more likely to be frank and explicit about expressing their sexual curiosity. Before or after his first wet dream, or even before puberty, a boy may learn that by hand he can stimulate his penis to erection and orgasm. Such stimulation is called **masturbation**. If he attempts this before puberty, he will have an orgasm without ejaculation, a powerful sensation that may be a strange combination of pain and pleasure. If he is sexually mature, he will simply find orgasm with ejaculation a brief and intense pleasure. For adolescent boys masturbation is a common and physically harmless act.

Girls and women, too, can masturbate, stimulating the clitoris to erection and orgasm, during which they will experience contractions of the vagina and wetness in the vagina and vulva, but no ejaculation. As with males, this is a physically harmless act.

Since masturbation has been the subject of severe disapproval in the past, and controversy now, I shall say more about it and its *consequences* later.

Completion of Puberty in the Male

Puberty continues, with the following developments: general body growth; **deepening of the voice**; a heavier moustache and the beginnings of a beard; coarser pubic and axillary hair; coarser hair on legs, arms, and chest. Meanwhile, the penis and testicles grow to adult size, and the rate of sperm production increases. The adult penis is on average 3 1/2 inches long when limp, 6 inches when erect. (The limp penis can shrink to half its normal length when a male feels chilly or nervous.) Mature testicles are about the size and shape of very large ripe olives. (Incidentally, it is quite normal for one testicle to hang lower than the other.) By the end of puberty the rate of sperm production has reached its peak: 40 million to 300 million in a single ejaculate from a mature, fertile male, even though the average amount of semen is approximately a teaspoonful.

There is no periodic shutdown in secretion of testosterone and other male hormones. Production of spermatozoa continues without interruption, a significant difference from the periodic menstrual cycle in women.

PSYCHOLOGICAL IMPLICATIONS OF ADOLESCENCE IN BOYS

Now as I did with girls on the subject of adolescence and menstruation, I must say more about the effects of adolescence on boys. As with girls, adolescence in boys begins with puberty and ends in adulthood, when the mature young man can mingle and compete comfortably with other adults. That may be as early as age 18 and as late as 24.

Differences in Maturation. Adolescence in boys is a time of differing rates of emotional, intellectual, and body change, in addition to sexual development. Boys who enter puberty earlier than their peers soon outstrip them in muscular development and in height. They also feel more mature than their prepubescent friends. They are in demand for competitive sports among older boys, and they are welcome in the company of older boys. This causes ruptures of friendships with less mature boys of the same age.

Among males, young and adult, such heavy emphasis is placed on muscular build and on manliness in sports that many pubescent boys feel tempted to act scornful toward their less developed male peers. This attitude makes teenage years particularly painful for boys who begin puberty later. Open shower and toilet facilities for males in schools, camps, and other institutions are invitations to comparisons. Falsetto imitations of boys whose voices haven't yet changed and locker-room taunts about undeveloped penis size are more hurtful than the tormentor may care to imagine.

Accepting Differences. Human society depends on sensitive respect of individuals for each other. It also depends on strength of character, and strength of character means a willingness to stand up as an individual and show respect and kindness, rather than going along with the crowd. Maturing boys should weigh the *consequences of cruelty* against the *consequences of kindness*. My hope is that they will reject temptations to tease and scorn the less developed among their peers and remember that biological development is mostly beyond control.

In addition to age differences in onset of puberty, there are differences in ways boys grow and develop during puberty. Some boys transform immediately into handsome young men. On the surface and to casual observers, this may seem wonderfully good luck, but it can have its disadvantages, as I shall point out later. Most, however, go through a temporary awkward stage, during which they are more angular and loose-jointed, or shorter or fatter or less muscular, than they wish to be. Many boys see their facial features growing out of proportion, and others are upset by acne. Some notice tenderness and lumpiness in the nipple area and also breast growth. Called **gynecomastia** (jin-e-koMASStia), this latter condition, not uncommon, must never be ridiculed. These sources of worry and embarrassment diminish during final stages of adolescence, but boys troubled by gynecomastia should tell their parents and seek advice from a physician.

In fact, in adolescent development every youth differs from every other youth, even after reaching full sexual maturity. Some young men have broad shoulders and muscular builds; others have lean, less muscular bodies; still others have a fuller distribution of fat. Chests vary: in shape from wide to barrel, in muscle mass from much to little, in nipple areola area from that of a quarter coin to that of a dime. Some young men have heavy beards, others light; some much body hair, others little. They differ also in density, coarseness, and distribution of pubic hair and in size of penis. Penis length may vary from the average an inch or more either way, limp or erect; and circumference too may vary. Penis and scrotum are usually darker than the surrounding skin, sometimes much darker.

Word for word as I have described for girls, some of the anxieties for boys are the same. For boys, too, a lively interest in studies, hobbies, and sports, and in organizations of service to other people, can do much to overcome these anxieties; and they are vital to the development of a youth's social and intellectual skills. Friends and strangers overlook all sorts of physical awkwardness when personality is outgoing and not *self*-conscious. These social and intellectual skills are especially important to youths who are awkward in sports, because males are brought up to value athletic prowess very heavily.

Sexual Urge and Maturing Intellect. While the physical changes of puberty are occurring, the sex hormones are also stimulating psychological changes. The pubescent boy feels mysteriously attracted to adolescent girls and boys and may discover they are attracted to him. He is curious about the development of his own body. His curiosity about sex intensifies. He may become infatuated with a particular girl, or, as happens with some boys, feel so sexually motivated that his peers may call him "horny." These psychological changes, part of the biological mechanisms that ensure sexual reproduction, are complex and stressful, however, so more about them in Part II.

Intellectual changes are also taking place. An adolescent boy discovers his ability to think abstractly about values and morals and ethics has greatly expanded. Since the *consequences* of the process of maturation depend on a youth's thinking about values and morals and ethics, I shall return to this theme later.

Sexual Self-knowledge
And Hygiene

In addition to the explanations already given in this book, girls and boys should be familiar with their own external genitalia. Girls should know how to keep clean and avoid urinary-tract and vaginal infections. Wiping after toilet use should be front to back, never back to front. Showers are preferable to tub baths. Cleaning of the vulva should be gentle, with a nonfragrant cleanser, and if a washrag is used instead of clean hands, the washcloth should be soft and clean, not left over from earlier bathing. Drying should be by patting gently with a clean towel or tissues. Daily change of clean cotton underwear is important. Talc powders are irritating, and gynecologists now recommend substitutes.   Use of a douche is to be discouraged; it washes out good bacteria that preserve the health of the vagina. Parents and phys-ed teachers should prepare prepubescent girls for menstruation and show how to use (and dispose of) absorbent pads and tampons. Commercial instructions accompanying packaging of tampons and absorbent pads are practical and helpful. *An adolescent girl should be able to talk freely about such things with her parents and with a gynecologist or family physician*; and she should immediately report any genital soreness and redness or unusual vaginal discharge or pelvic pain.

Self-diagnosis for discomfort or infection is dangerous, and over-the-counter medication of the genitalia should never be used without a physician's diagnosis and advice.

Boys should keep their genitals clean. Uncircumcised boys should pull back their foreskins when bathing, to clean between the fold of skin and the head of the penis. Otherwise, secretions form a cheese-like, irritating deposit (smegma) that can cause infection. Ordinarily, foreskins are loose enough to be pulled back easily. If not, they are usually loosened by medical or surgical means. One should not attempt to force back the tight skin. Boys should be familiar with the feel of their testicles and the epididymal mass attached to each testicle. Hand examination is best done after a warm bath or shower, when the testicles hang low in the scrotum. Importance of this has to do with the rare occurrence of testicular cancer in youths, and adults too. Discovery of an unexpected lump, usually hard, should be reported immediately. So should testicular pain. And in contact sports and games involving flying pucks and balls, boys should wear jockstraps and/or plastic cups. *Boys should feel as free to talk with parents and family doctors about genital health concerns and problems as about other health problems or worries.*

Health and the Marketing of Sex

Overemphasis on physical attractiveness has created physical as well as psychological health hazards to growing into productive adulthood. Earlier in this text, you may recall, I devoted considerable space (some in small print) to endocrine glands and their secretions, all of which are in delicate balance as they affect our growth, development, and sexual maturation. Endocrinologists traditionally warn that untested (and even tested) experimentation and treatment with hormones can lead to harmful imbalances. Unfortunately---disastrously, in my opinion---the sports industry and the male beauty industry have promoted use of anabolic steroids (which are synthetic hormones) to increase muscular bulk and athletic performance. Though use of these steroids is banned, unscrupulous dealers make

34

them available, and boys and adolescents (especially body builders and serious athletes) use them to build glamorous bodies and to create unfair advantage in athletic competition. Temptations to use these steroids must be weighed against subsequent harmful effects. By throwing normal secretions of hormones off balance, users risk not only a lasting change in normal growth and development but also long-range damage to such vital organs as liver, heart, and kidneys---not to mention reproductive organs. Psychological damage is equally disastrous; once a youth loves his bulked musculature, he desires more and begins to believe his mirrored image is inadequate---bodybuilder's "anorexia." Emotional and personality damage is also a consequence, which can destroy family relations.

By the way, forced weight gain or loss to "make the team" can be equally harmful.

Girls too are targets of unscrupulous marketing of hormonal enhancements of body beauty and development. Ads for creams and ointments with hormone additives boast of clearing blemishes from skin. Unscrupulous merchants (and sometimes coaches) illegally promote anabolic steroids for advantage in athletic competition. Anabolic steroids masculinize musculature and interfere with natural development of the female body. They interfere with the menstrual cycle and cause long-range harm to health, including risks of cancer and strokes. Another health hazard is use of herbal compounds in pill form, supposedly to increase breast size. Aside from unproven cosmetic results, these compounds can react dangerously with prescribed medicines.

There is now a new physical danger: cosmetic surgery---liposuction and injection of silicon gels to sculpture the body, beautification measures taken to absurd extremes.

Perhaps the most insidious threat to an adolescent girl's health---for the sake of attractiveness---is weight loss. Female models for clothing and cosmetics are almost skeletal in thinness. Somehow this has become a standard for what the advertising industry and entertainment industry consider attractiveness. And see how the pharmaceutical industry has capitalized on this to sell weight-loss programs and pills! One tragic consequence of this slenderizing obsession can be a shut-down of vital organ function. Another is the life-threatening psychological disease of anorexia or bulimia.

You may recall my earlier statement that the boy who grows naturally into the idealized model of handsome youth, or the girl who grows naturally into the idealized model of glamorous beauty, may not be so lucky. Here's why. Such attractiveness---biologically ideal for sexual attraction---places a premium on physical beauty, sometimes to the exclusion of personality and character development. When personality development and character development are neglected, the instant popularity of handsomeness and beauty disappears with the bloom of youth But let it be said: handsome youths and beautiful young women whose developing personalities and characters have saved them from self-absorption are lucky indeed.

As I have stated throughout this book, the advertising and entertainment industries spend millions of dollars on sexual enticement, and the return is in billions. Sex sells, but when it is irresponsibly and exploitively peddled, the consequences are hazardous to health and cheapening to our most intimate interpersonal relationships.

A Biological Imperative:
Sexual Intercourse

Since reproduction is essential to the survival of species, and since human beings reproduce sexually, the act of **sexual intercourse** is a biological imperative. I write *a* biological imperative because the evolution of human beings as a species with intellectual powers enables us to enjoy our lives in other dimensions quite special to us in addition to the reproductive imperative. While other species reproduce compulsively and have complex and apparently inborn means of nurturing their young, we---with our intellect---could not survive in such a way. In addition to our sexual drive (which is literally programmed into us by DNA, as it is in other life forms), we have the capacity for discovering beauty and for creating and appreciating all the arts; we delight in physical and intellectual games; we have an apparently innate sense of justice, from which develop conscience and moral and ethical values; and we are capable of deep commitments to friendships and to those we love. These, too, are biological imperatives for *our* survival. They develop from our ability to reason and to think in the abstract. I shall show you, from time to time in these pages, how these other imperatives are a part of our understanding of *sex and consequences*.

The act which initiates reproduction in mammals, the class to which we belong, is also called **copulation** or **mating** or **coitus** (COitus).

"Having sex," now in common usage, is an expression I find offensive because it devalues the act as well as the accepted grammar of biology. I use the term **sexual intercourse** because it is widely accepted and because it expresses the idea of mutual spoken consent between two intelligent people.

Under ideal circumstances, sexual intercourse is the ultimate act of love and trust between husband and wife, and it is therefore often called **making love**, perhaps an even better expression. In these ideal circumstances, there is nothing furtive, no feeling of guilt; only joy and pleasure in the intimate caressing and embracing of **foreplay** that arouses the couple to seek climax in physical and emotional intercourse.

Like most human activities, however, sexual intercourse needs learning. First attempts may be embarrassingly clumsy, even painful, and therefore require patience, sensitivity to each other's feelings, and a sense of humor---attributes of adult maturity. These are among the reasons, discussed later, why many young people seriously consider abstaining from sexual intercourse until such mature commitment as marriage.

Conception. Immediately after ejaculation in sexual intercourse, the spermatozoa swim into the uterus and toward the oviducts. No one knows precisely what chemical and physical stimuli direct the spermatozoa, but *if ovulation has occurred within the 24-36 hours before intercourse*, one spermatozoon, out of the tens of thousands that enter each oviduct, *may* penetrate the one mature ovum descending one of the two tubes. And thus begins **conception**, or **fertilization**, the addition of the sperm's half of genetic material to the egg's half, to initiate a potential new life.

This concludes Part I, which has taken you through the biology and some of the psychology and consequences of sexually coming of age. Part II explores what is meant by sexuality and its psychological and social consequences.

PART II

Sexuality, And Its Effects On
The Imperative Of Sexual Intercourse

DISCOVERING YOUR SEXUALITY

You may remember that the parents' genes in the fertilized egg determine whether an offspring will be male or female. More complicated are the *personal characteristics* of the two sexes---masculinity of appearance and behavior in males, femininity of appearance and behavior in females; more commonly, mixtures of these characteristics in either sex. These characteristics we call the **sexuality** of the individual. *Sexuality* is determined partly by the genetic makeup of a person. It is also determined by the balance of hormones in the maternal blood while the embryo develops in the womb, and by the balance of hormones in the blood of the developing offspring after birth. It is also affected by social conditioning. From the moment of an infant's birth, parents and all the instruments of society direct, program, and condition that infant's behavior and expectations toward standards of sexuality thought to be consistent with the infant's sex.

A vital part of boys' and girls' social development, especially during adolescence, is in discovering their *sexuality* and understanding the *consequences* of each new phase of this discovery. It is in every sense a learning experience. During puberty girls and boys become very conscious of their own and each others' appearance and behavior. Clothing, hair style, posture; patterns of speech and walking; interest in music, dance, sports; admiration for some of the stars of music, TV, movies, theater, and sports: these are just a few of the signals by which pubescent boys and girls try to attract, and are attracted to, each other. These signals are for members of the same sex as well as for members of the opposite sex. If a boy is accepted by peers of the same sex, he will probably be attractive to peers of the opposite sex. The same is true for girls.

Desires and needs to be attractive put tremendous pressures on youths to conform to the standards of acceptance of friends and would-be friends. With increasing insistence and intensity, the industries of fashion, recreation, entertainment, communications, and food and drink are stimulating and inducing young people to conform to each new trend. Commercial empires are built upon the sure knowledge that teenagers fear exclusion from their peers and will buy and imitate whatever it takes to be "in." People who understand this commercial motive call it "exploitation of the young."

Against this commercial drumbeat and the fast pace of in-school and outside activities and commitments, teenagers have less and less quiet time, by themselves or with family and a few very close friends, to discover who and what they really are. In quiet time each person---child, youth, or adult---sheds the customs of social interplay (some of which are pretense and some of which are genuine) to face the uncertainties of the inner self.

Discovery and management of the sexual self---alone and in social context---is the subject of these next few pages.

SOCIETAL AND PUBERTAL INFLUENCES ON GIRLS' SEXUALITY

Genetic factors responsible for inborn traits, including temperament, may have as much to do with expressions of girls' sexuality as do the external factors that follow.

Societal. From the moment of birth, a baby girl is treated like a "girl." In Western civilizations, as in the United States, hospitals identify infant girls with pink. Adults speak gently and cooingly to baby girls. Parents decorate girls' bedrooms with flower patterns and decorative draperies. Toys, after rattles and floating baubles, are likely to be dolls. Adults are amused by little girls' trying on their mothers' dresses, accessories, and makeup. They praise girls for grace in stance and motion. They discourage boyish aggressiveness and yield to girls' emotional persuasions. A girl's tears evoke more sympathy than contempt.

And there are the role models, peer pressures, and commercial entertainments. For little girls the models are the cartoon flirtations of seductive birds, fish, mermaids, and caricatured human females. For prepubescent girls, cliques in school degrade boys and shun girls who don't fit the popular mold, and models outside school are teeniebopper song-and-dance stars who invite daring in dress and language. For pubescent girls the models are slender, scantily clad starlets---coyly or brazenly enticing---in teen magazines, TV commercials and daytime dramas, and the much more explicitly vulgar MTV. Seductive and daring songs, commercials, and sitcoms tell girls what boys "expect of them." Sitcoms and daytime dramas make sexual intercourse casual and expected.

To counterbalance these commercial influences (in which millions of dollars are invested), parents, schools, and religious institutions struggle to recognize and reward good role models from among girls' teachers and counselors and especially from among girls' most responsible and sensitive peers.

Though current trends in bringing up girls allow and encourage greater opportunity for education and competition in what were once the preserves of boys and men, traditional pressures for exclusively "feminine" interests and activities are everywhere pervasive. External society's expectations of what a girl and woman should be are powerful forces, regardless of how thoughtfully parents try to prepare their daughters to express the wonderful variety of their individual personalities.

Pubertal. At puberty, when hormones stimulate increased sexual curiosity and attraction, girls' hopes and desires are strongly affected by romantic images acquired during childhood development. Thus sexual curiosity is more likely to be satisfied through romantic involvement than by sexual experimentation just for the sake of experimentation. Even experimental masturbation is likely to be accompanied by romantic fantasies and the wish for shared romantic and sexual experience. Yearning to nurture and to become a mother seems biologically inherent, but that yearning may be in deep conflict with desire for, and growing commitment to, the goal of a rewarding career.

Societal and Pubertal, Together. During this pubertal time, a girl's thoughts may be thronged with conflicting dreams and apprehensions. Will she fit the slender, full-breasted model so compellingly and commercially presented as lures for boys? Should she diet to fit the model? Is she "feminine" enough? Is she "boy crazy"? Is she too little attracted to boys? Is the affection she has for another girl something to worry about? How different from her feelings about boys are boys' feelings about her? How flirtatious, accessible, even aggressive should she be to attract a boy? What do boys expect of her, and how should she respond? *What are the consequences of exploring these questions?*

The suddenly increased biological imperative of sexual curiosity and attraction during puberty is expressed through and beyond the sexual identity established in a girl's earlier years. The cumulative effect, by the end of adolescence, defines the sexuality of the young woman. One's developing sexuality and its consequences will be discussed later. Lucky is the girl who can grow up comfortably inside her changing body while affected by genes and hormones and socially conditioned by the challenges of changing norms.

SOCIETAL AND PUBERTAL INFLUENCES ON BOYS' SEXUALITY

Genetic factors responsible for inborn traits, including temperament, may have as much to do with expressions of boys' sexuality as do the external factors that follow.

Societal. From birth a baby boy is treated like a "boy." Hospitals identify a male infant with blue. He is held more playfully, less gently than a baby girl. At home his crib sheets and bedroom are likely to be decorated, if at all, with pictures of cowboys, sailboats, animals. Early graduation to short pants and a boy's haircut is a major establishment of masculinity. Toys are likely to be balls, puzzles, construction blocks, toy guns and trucks, mechanical gadgets, and computer games involving violent pursuit. The boy can try on Daddy's shoes but not Mommy's clothes and accessories. Adults discourage so-called feminine grace and encourage athletic skills and sports. They praise aggressive self-assertion and teach skills in running, jumping, climbing, and tussling. They treat tears with contempt rather than sympathy.

Popular but desensitizing role models for little boys are the daring boy heroes of Saturday TV cartoons and, later, the gun-toting superman dolls and muscle-bound superheroes of comic books and computerized games. For older boys, the models are teenage athletes and the shoot-em-up musclemen of violent movies. In school, peers encourage prepubescent boys to swagger aggressively and to ignore or harass girls. Boys dare not show interest in girls' conversations and activities lest they be called sissies or faggots. For adolescent boys, role models are professional athletes and the crude and sexually aggressive singers and dancers of rock bands and MTV. Magazine ads and TV commercials, especially those promoting soft drinks and beer, portray young males as handsome rogues seeking seductive young females as sex objects. Daytime and evening TV dramas do the same, often adding physical and verbal abuse to relationships and making sexual intercourse seem a casual and to-be-expected sport.

To counterbalance these influences, parents, school teachers and administrators, and religious institutions struggle to reward good role models from among boys' teachers and counselors and especially from among boys' most responsible and sensitive peers.

Though today's trends in bringing up boys allow and encourage greater opportunity for education and competition in what were once only for girls and women, traditional pressures for self-assertion, male dominance, and athletic prowess are all around us. Society's expectations are powerful forces, no matter how thoughtfully parents try to prepare their sons to express the variety of their individual personalities.

Pubertal. At puberty, when hormones stimulate sexual curiosity and attraction, the youthful boy's daydreams and desires are strongly affected by fantasies of romance and sexual fulfillment. As sexual curiosity intensifies, it usually leads to sexual experimentation, masturbation being the most common, followed by attempts to discover shared romantic and sexual experience. In the background is hope for marriage and the raising of a family, but the drive for explicitly sexual activity is more immediately urgent.

Societal and Pubertal, Together. During this time of development, a boy's thoughts may be thronged with conflicting hopes and apprehensions. Will he fit the bulked-up muscular model so admired by his peers and so attractive to girls? Is he "masculine" enough? Is he too consumed with sexual desire? Is he "girl crazy"? Is he too little attracted to girls? Does he masturbate too frequently? Is the attraction he feels for another boy something to worry about? How different from his feelings about girls are girls' feelings about him? How aggressive or reticent should he be in his sexual experimentation? What do girls expect of him sexually and romantically, and how should he respond? *What are the consequences of exploring these questions?*

The biological imperative of sexual curiosity and attraction during puberty is expressed through and beyond the sexual identity established in a boy's earlier years. The cumulative effect, by the end of adolescence, defines the sexuality of the young man.

DISCOVERING YOUR SEXUAL ORIENTATION

Among questions pubescent boys and girls have about their sexuality is their curiosity about their **sexual orientation** and the consequences of that orientation. Sexual orientation refers to the nature in which a person feels sexually attracted. In examining and discussing sexual orientation, we must try to understand what characteristics of sexuality can be modified and what cannot, and then we must learn how to understand what *expressions* of sexuality are socially responsible and what are not.

Heterosexuality.   The prefix *hetero-* comes from the Greek word *heteros*, meaning *the other* or *the different* of two.   The adjective **heterosexual** means *sexually attracted by, and to, the opposite sex.* Most human beings are sexually attracted to members of the opposite sex. They are said to be **heterosexually oriented**.   The genetic and hormonal makeup of the developing fetus tends to ensure heterosexuality.   So also do the mother's hormones affect the fetus.   And the later conditioning by parents and society plays a role.   Thus the great majority of boys are sexually attracted to girls, and vice versa, and this attraction continues from childhood through adolescence and maturity into old age.   Such attraction is, obviously, vital to the survival of our species.

Within the heterosexual population, however, as among other mammals, there is much variety.   Many heterosexuals are exclusively heterosexual; they are sexually attracted only to people of the opposite sex.   This doesn't mean that exclusively heterosexual people don't admire and appreciate physical beauty in people of the same sex, and it doesn't mean they don't have close friendships with people of the same sex.   It means they are *sexually* drawn only to people of the *opposite* sex.   Even their sexual fantasies and sexual dreams are almost always exclusively heterosexual.

Other heterosexuals may sometimes feel attracted sexually to members of the same sex.   This may be temporary, as a part of adolescent development, or a continuing mild-to-strong attraction despite basically heterosexual orientation.   Their sexual fantasies and sexual dreams, though usually heterosexual, may also involve same-sex attraction,

Homosexuality.   The prefix *homo-* comes from the Greek word *homo*, which means *same* (not to be confused with the Latin *homo*, which means *human*, as in our biological name, Homo sapiens or *wise human*).   **Homosexuality** is sexual attraction to members of the same sex.   People who are more attracted to members of the same sex than the opposite sex are said to be **homosexually oriented**.   Biological studies of sexual behavior among humans and other primates include homosexuality within the normal range of sexual orientation.   Genetic and hormonal factors seem to be major determiners of homosexuality, as they are of heterosexuality.

47

Some people are exclusively homosexual, sexually attracted only to people of the same sex. Though they are not sexually attracted to members of the opposite sex, they are just as capable as heterosexuals of having strong and lasting friendships with members of the opposite sex. Conditioning by parents and society seems to have no counterdetermining effect on exclusively homosexual orientation. I use the words *seem* and *seems* because a few psychologists and behavioral scientists claim success in reversing homosexuality, but such success is questionable. Statistical studies of homosexuality suggest that about 2-3 per cent of the population is exclusively homosexual. The sexual fantasies and sexual dreams of exclusively homosexual people are almost always exclusively homosexual.

As with heterosexuals, there is variation in homosexual orientation. Many homosexuals are somewhat attracted sexually to members of the opposite sex. This may be occasional or it may be an ongoing mild-to-strong attraction despite a basic homosexual orientation. People with such divided sexual attraction have sexual fantasies and sexual dreams that are usually homosexual though occasionally heterosexual. Such orientation may be found among as much as 5 percent of the population, in addition to the exclusively homosexual. As I stated above, conditioning by parents and society seems to have little counterdetermining effect on homosexual attraction.

Bisexuality. Some people feel equally drawn sexually to members of either sex, and they prefer to be called **bisexual**.

Transvestism. Cross-dressing. People with an overwhelming desire to wear clothes of the opposite sex are called **transvestites**. They are likely to be heterosexual males.

Transsexualism. A few people feel intensely that they should be of the opposite sex. A boy or man may feel so strongly that he should be a girl or woman that he is willing to dress accordingly and even undergo surgery and hormone treatment to simulate the change of sex. Similarly, a girl or woman may feel just as strongly that she should be a boy or man. People with this intense and irreconcilable desire call themselves **transsexuals** (often the euphemistic **transgenders**). After adopting the dress, behavior, and customs of the opposite sex, many transsexuals live satisfactory lives.

Straight, Gay, Lesbian, and Bi. These are politically correct terms used in discussions of sexual orientation. "Straight" refers to heterosexuality; "gay" refers to homosexuality in general but usually male; "lesbian" refers to female homosexuality; and "bi" refers to bisexuality. The word *lesbian*, by the way, comes from the Greek island Lesbos, where the 6th-century B.C. poet Sappho lived and wrote her famous poems of lust and love. Her women admirers and disciples were referred to as Lesbians.

SOCIAL ATTITUDES
TOWARD SEXUAL ORIENTATION

Human society in its varying cultures has varying attitudes toward the perceived sexuality of its members. Regardless of what anthropologists, psychologists, and sociologists may say is within the normal range of sexual orientation, society in general (certainly in the United States) accepts heterosexual orientation most positively and without question. People belonging to a statistically very large majority feel unchallenged in that majority and assume others feel and act as they do. Heterosexuals assume everyone else is heterosexual unless they discover or are informed otherwise. The "otherwise" is what causes problems.

To discuss the *otherwise*, let's first look at some parallels or analogies, cautioned, however, that analogies don't fit in every respect. Among gatherings of people who don't know each other well, there are three topics we politely agree not to discuss: religion, politics, and sex. These are topics that nearly everyone takes personally and seriously. We know not to speak or act offensively about religions that differ from our own. We shouldn't force our religious beliefs or nonbeliefs on others, and we resent having others' beliefs or nonbeliefs forced on us. So too with politics. However happily or unhappily we accept the will of the majority at the polls, we don't like to hear our political convictions attacked at a gathering of people who aren't polite enough to sense our feelings. And so too with sex. People with sexual orientations different from our own can be terribly hurt or angered if we question or speak or act disparagingly about their orientation, just as we feel if our own sexual orientation is questioned or attacked.

Though homosexuality is within the normal range of sexual orientation, it is generally looked upon as "out of the ordinary." Because it doesn't fulfill ordinary expectations of heterosexual dating, marriage, procreation, and child rearing, it raises fears, especially among parents and other guardians of standard behavior. Since causes of homosexuality are not fully known, and same-sex attraction is apparently beyond the ability of the homosexual to change, fear of homosexuality produces strong social attitudes that can be harmful to individuals and troubling to various institutions of society. Pre-adolescents and adolescents who feel sexually drawn to people of the same sex may become terrified of their personal development and of being discovered. Some peers may avoid associating with those who fit society's stereotype of homosexuality for fear of being themselves labeled and ridiculed as "queer" or "gay." Such fears, though based in part on ignorance, can lead to hostility, hatred, and violence.

Added to these fears of "out of the ordinary" sexual orientation are other problems for homosexuals: religious restrictions, military service restrictions, and AIDS. Several religions regard homosexual activity as sinful, citing scripture as authority. Elders, priests, and preachers of these religions may accept homosexuals lovingly, but forbid engagement in homosexual acts. And now there is the danger of AIDS, a disease most frequently transmitted by careless sexual activity, diagnosed first among actively homosexual males in the early 1980s and now spreading among drug users and heterosexual males and females. Public association of AIDS with homosexuality is one more burden that a young person who suspects he is homosexual must bear. Thus the vital importance of compassion and available counseling for young people worried about their sexuality. And thus the importance of being socially accepting of homosexuals as being like all of us, with our differences and similarities.

I shall deal with AIDS later in connection with sexually transmitted diseases. Meanwhile, stereotypes in appearance and behavior among heterosexual and homosexual males and females will be a part of the next section. But right now I remind you that knowledge of consequences, combined with a well-developed sense of responsibility, can do much to relieve fears and to encourage happy lives.

DEALING WITH STEREOTYPES IN SEXUAL ORIENTATION

At puberty, when hormonal changes intensify sexual curiosity, self-experimentation and social experimentation gradually lead to self-awareness of sexual orientation. Many young adolescents feel no doubt of their basic heterosexuality and soon project images of assurance and comfort with heterosexuality in themselves and in others. They fit the most commonly perceived *stereotypes* of heterosexuality. A **stereotype** is what the public has learned to accept as a pattern of looks and behavior typical of a group. As an example, television commercials for soft drinks and beer present exaggerated (and potentially harmful) stereotypes of young heterosexual males and females.

The stereotype, however, is often not the reality. Many heterosexual adolescents lack the carefree social mannerisms glorified in commercials. Some strive, sometimes successfully, to emulate these models. Others, feeling less pressure to conform, don't care to emulate. But many, though sure of their basic heterosexuality, are distressed by their inability to fit the mold or stereotype.

The greatest pressure is on adolescents who are unsure of their sexual orientation or who know they are homosexual. Stereotypes of male and female homosexuals are presented exaggeratedly in movies and TV, so I need not describe them here any more than the stereotypes of heterosexuals. Fearful of taunts by peers and adults, many adolescent homosexuals try to adopt the stereotypical images of heterosexuals, often so successfully that they escape the cruelties that careless and irresponsible heterosexuals would inflict upon them, and they avoid situations that would require heterosexual intimacy. Other adolescent homosexuals, unable to adopt the heterosexual stereotypes, isolate themselves from social situations in which they might feel exposed, or they openly admit to their orientation ("come out of the closet," so to speak). In either case their suffering is acute, though less so nowadays as society becomes more and more accepting of differences in orientation (see pages 58-59).

Before discussing responsible behavior and attitudes, I want to make the point that "you can't judge a book by its cover." Some heterosexuals fit the homosexual stereotype in looks, interests, and manner. Some homosexuals fit the heterosexual stereotype in looks, interests, and manner. It is unrealistic to presume sexual orientation on the basis of appearance.

Manifesting Sexuality
Through Expression and Behavior

Expression. As in all other human transactions, expression of sexuality and sexual desire should be respectful of the feelings and privacy of others, especially because it is basic to the most intensely personal and emotionally vulnerable part of our being. Despite irresponsible display of sex-without-consequences in TV shows and movies, there is growing concern among adults and adolescents that there should be boundaries to sexual behavior. Let's look first at generally accepted codes and manners for *expressing sexuality*, then generally accepted codes and manners in *sexual behavior*.

"Generally accepted by whom or what?" you might ask. By family, school, religious institutions, doctors and psychologists, political institutions, and the law---all the people and institutions that make for a civil and responsible society. This is not to say that such codes and manners do not change with time and knowledge, but the customs of civilization reside in these people and institutions.

Heterosexual Expression. Among pubescent students in coeducational classrooms, the earlier tendency of boys and girls to sit apart breaks down, and one sees a girl seeking a seat next to a boy or vice versa, almost a territorial expression of sexuality. Of course, good friends of the same sex continue to pick out seats next to each other, but heterosexual attraction sometimes disrupts old friendships. Disruption of old friendships is a consequence of puberty that one should be aware of and make a conscious effort to modify; not easy when a boy's girl friend or a girl's boy friend is jealous of old friendship ties. Development of social sensitivity, however, is a part of responsible behavior in growing up.

Expression of heterosexual attraction then progresses to "dating" behavior, which has varied so much from generation to generation, region to region, culture to culture, and fad to fad that I can only define it as the complex of strategies that heterosexual boys and girls use to express their desire to be in each other's company. It was once the custom of the boy to take the lead in expressing his interest in a particular girl. Nowadays girls are just as likely to take the lead. First efforts are most successful when they are as casual and simply friendly as possible. Intensity usually results in awkwardness that can lead to embarrassment. Casual and friendly situations and circumstances provide the easiest opportunities for expression.

Respect for the other person's feelings and dignity is vital to an adolescent's healthy and happy expression of sexual attraction. So is respect for that person's parents and one's own parents. Parents are naturally protective of their children. Having gone through their own temptations, dangers, and disappointments while growing up, they need to know, and should know, that their youthful offspring are among respectful and respectable companions. A mutually respectful and lasting relationship is most likely to develop from similar interests and similar participation in cultural, social, and athletic events. This is the kind of relationship that responsible parents encourage and which young adolescents find most congenial and least troublesome.

What do responsible parents worry about as being unacceptable or undesirable heterosexual expression among their young adolescents? Young adolescent couples alone and unsupervised; young adolescents at unsupervised parties. In both kinds of circumstances, temptations are elevated for sexual experimentation that can lead to unanticipated and unhappy consequences.

Much as teenagers seek independence from parents, they really respect, even long for, parental caring and guidance. Subconsciously they hope their parents want to know what they are up to. A responsible teenage boy and teenage girl can easily be respectful of each other when a responsible parent is nearby, but with unsupervised groups and couples the tendency to show off can lead to insensitivity. Boys and girls in groups may think it's exciting to dare each other with sexually suggestive comments that can quickly escalate into crudeness and harassment, sometimes even physical, such as touching or grabbing breasts and genitals. Such irresponsible group behavior is totally degrading to a girl's and boy's sense of inner worth and self-respect. But it takes only one or two brave people to speak up and put others to shame for behaving this way.

Also to be avoided are relationships based solely on sexual attraction, with sexual activity (currently called "hooking up") being the only goal, usually for the boy with no reciprocal pleasure for the girl. Such relationships are short lived and quickly disrespectful, often to the distress of the girl, who can feel used, abused, and abandoned. And especially to be avoided are romantic relationships in which the two are significantly different in age or in sexual maturity and sexual experience. The older or more mature person may be seeking conquest by seduction---finding special pleasure in taking away the other's sexual innocence. Obviously, if *you* are the older, more experienced person, you must avoid being the seducer. Ways of handling these situations are in Part IV.

Moreover, and vitally important, be extremely wary of sexual encounters via the Internet, some of which can turn out to be with literally murderous predators. More about this later (see pages 58 and 74).

The most positive and healthy heterosexual relationships are long lasting in friendship, ones that grow in understanding, respect, and **fidelity** (faithfulness) to one another. The most destructive and unhealthy heterosexual relationships are based on **promiscuity**; that is, seeking and giving oneself sexually to one partner after another without regard for bonds of respect, mutual interests, and the inner person.

Homosexual Expression. Imagine how much more awkward, indeed isolating and frightening, it is for homosexual youths to try to express their affection for, and attraction to, each other. We are supposedly more tolerant of gays and lesbians than we were several generations ago, but the kinds of male-to-male friendships and female-to-female friendships that were idealized as wholesome and good a hundred years ago are now looked on with suspicion, as though they *must* be *sexual*. Today we tend to label people by religion, nationality, race, ethnicity, politics, and sexual orientation---a characteristic that dehumanizes the respectable person underneath. So we hear young people making such hurtful comments as, "What a faggot!" or, "He's so gay!" or, "She's such a dyke!"

And if the boy *is* gay or suspects he is, and the girl *is* lesbian or suspects she is, what an unhappy time that young person has in seeking the affections that heterosexuals so openly express! Adolescents are especially concerned about their sexuality and about their parents' and society's hopes and expectations and about their peers' reactions to their expressions of sexuality. A gay boy's or a gay girl's attempt to look at or talk flirtatiously with someone of the same sex---as heterosexual boys and girls so easily do with each other---risks instant labeling of self and possibly of the other person. Beyond that, and especially among boys, the reaction can be violent.

What are homosexual adolescents to do in seeking some expression of romantic yearnings? Be respectful, observant, cautious. Sensitivity to the dignity and reputations of one's fellow human beings is the basis of respectfulness. Awareness of other people's interests and talents---cultural, social, and physical---is vital to being observant. Caution and courtesy are the common sense in then approaching the other person in a conversationally intimate manner. Feelings of compatibility between two homosexual people usually develop in such ways, allowing the beginning of a lasting, mutually satisfying, responsible friendship, *the positive consequence of ethical sexual behavior.*

Schools, colleges, and society in general are beginning to recognize gay and lesbian students' need to socialize in a manner accepting of their sexuality, thus encouraging open, healthy relationships among straights and gays and reducing secrecy and furtiveness. Professional counseling from responsible adults associated with gay/straight alliances also encourages healthy relationships and can assist young people in the difficult decision of opening themselves to their parents. I hope this book, too, will be helpful in creating understanding and compassion about differing sexual orientations.

And what are homosexual adolescents to avoid in seeking expression of their sexuality? Seduction, victimization, promiscuity. Here are some "don'ts." Don't approach a person with seduction as your goal (don't lure that person for sexual gratification), and don't victimize a person as a subject of your sexual desires. Don't seek romantic friendship with a younger, more innocent person. Don't yield your innocence to someone seeking your friendship only for sexual gratification. Avoid advances of an older, more sexually experienced person, or a person your age but more mature and experienced. Don't tempt adults. Avoid friendships based only on sexual gratification. Ways of handling these situations are discussed in Part IV.

Avoid **promiscuity**; that is, partner after partner, sexual gratification the only incentive, without regard for bonds of respect, mutual interests, and the inner person. And be extremely wary of encounters via the Internet, some of which can turn out to be with literally murderous predators. More about this later (see page 74).

The most destructive, unhealthy homosexual relationships are based on promiscuity. Unfortunately, societal suspicions of homosexuality, especially male, make it difficult to find responsible, respectable homosexual friends and to sustain long-lasting relationships. This societal attitude encourages furtive, brief, and risky encounters.

Seek **fidelity**, faithfulness to one another. The most positive and healthy homosexual and heterosexual relationships are long lasting---ones that grow in understanding, respect, love, and fidelity to one another. Fortunately, social and legal customs are more and more encouraging of long-lasting and faithful homosexual relationships, recognizing loving partnership bonding and, in some jurisdictions, marital status.

The genetic urge to have children and to rear them lovingly and responsibly is not restricted to heterosexuals. Homosexuals living together in faithful and trusting relationships have legal rights in some states to adopt children. And some lesbian couples have brought children to their union through impregnation by artificial insemination from a sperm donor.

PART III

Social Imperatives

LOVE, SEX, AND HISTORY

Dating behavior, whether heterosexual or homosexual, may lead to conversational, emotional, and physical intimacies that are temptations to sexual intercourse. This makes do's and don't's more complicated. Here a clear sense of responsibility and respect, and a full understanding of consequences, is essential to moral judgment and conduct.

You will have noticed that I began my description of sexual intercourse (page 38) with the words "under ideal circumstances." These ideal circumstances involve extremely important social and personal responsibilities and consequences. To explain these responsibilities and consequences, I must discuss some social imperatives that are linked historically with the biological imperative.

In reading literature and other accounts of life in past centuries, we discover a history of changing customs and attitudes about sex, sexuality, and family life. In different times and cultures in the Western world, the appropriate age for marriage and having children has varied from early adolescence to mid-thirties. Family structure and economic conditions have always been important determinants. So also have been values systems of religions, cultures, and philosophies. And until the mid-1950s, fear of producing unwanted children was a primary deterrent to sexual intercourse outside marriage.

Among primates, the order of mammals to which we belong, puberty is the time for first attempts at mating. Among humans sexual maturation leads inevitably toward desire for sexual intercourse. From a strictly biological point of view, young post-adolescent couples who are bonded to each other by strong ties of love and lasting responsibility have been best suited to the special responsibilities of parenthood. This is when women and men are most attractive. Muscle and skin tone, fullness of lips, long eyelashes are at their peak for sexual attraction. Bodies are strongest, healthiest, and most resilient. And it is also a time when a woman can most effectively endure the stresses of childbirth and motherhood and a man can most effectively meet the challenges of fatherhood.

Complexities of living, however, have often discouraged marriage and childbearing until couples are in their middle twenties and early thirties, and that is true again today. But improved diet and other health conditions in the last fifty years have resulted in earlier sexual maturity; and in the 1950s a so-called *sexual revolution promoted increased sexual activity* among adolescents as well as among adults.

Because circumstances today require postponement of childbearing during the very years when you would be sexually most active, you and I should examine the religious, societal, medical, and philosophical factors that adolescents will find consequential when making decisions about love and sexual activity.

Historical Factors in Sexual Decision Making

Restraints

Until the 1950s the bonds that held 20th-century families together were much stronger than they are now. Religious institutions, schools, and parents preached commitment to sexual restraint, family loyalty, and marital fidelity (faithfulness to one's partner in marriage). Federal and state laws prohibited public displays of, and access to, sexually provocative information and activities. The entertainment industry and publishers were self-censoring. There were several reasons for this.

Religious Conviction. The Commandment "Thou shalt not commit adultery" means narrowly that sexual intercourse with any partner except one's spouse is morally wrong. Several religious sects interpret this commandment more broadly, preaching that any sexual activity outside marriage is sinful; and a few preach that *lust*---sexual desire and sexual activity solely for the sake of sexual pleasure, even in marriage---is sinful. Thus masturbation and other sexual activities that do not lead to procreation (conception and the creation of children) are similarly sinful. Children and adults brought up in this tradition are taught that such behavior can isolate one from God's love, even condemn one to hellfire. They are also taught that sexual pleasure is God's gift for the sole purpose of producing offspring among married couples. These are stern lessons, and they have had a powerful effect on many generations among Western civilizations.

Here I should write of current thinking about masturbation. Masturbation has long been thought of as sinful and harmful for boys and men; sinful because it "wastes the male seed," intended only for procreation, harmful because loss of male "vital fluid" was thought to weaken body and mind. It has also been thought of as sinful and harmful for girls and women, though there is no "loss of seed." Today, however, we are enlightened enough to know masturbation is not harmful, either physically or emotionally. Whether or not it is sinful depends on one's religious upbringing. Some religions continue to label it a sin; others no longer do.

Masturbation remains a subject of controversy, as you can read or hear in the media. In fact, public opinion is so divided on the subject that discussion of it quickly becomes heated, a consequence one should be aware of in conversations. Here, however, is current medical and psychological opinion. Practiced alone and in privacy, it is *safe from disease*, a harmless, pleasurable way of learning about sexual arousal and orgasm. As a solitary act, its pleasure, however, is an end in itself. How frequently one masturbates depends on frequency and intensity of urge and on self-control. Self-control in sexual behavior is as important to character and self-esteem as is self-control in other patterns of behavior. (See pages 29, 72, 75, 79-80, 98 for further discussion of masturbation.)

Fear of Pregnancy out of Wedlock. Until the 20th-century sexual revolution (which I will describe later), an unwed pregnant girl or woman was shamed and scorned, subjected to expulsion from school or college or workplace, sometimes even from her home. Parents of adolescent girls, fearful of these social consequences and respectful of religious and moral strictures against adulterous behavior, put the burden of sexual restraint on their daughters. And they were strongly supported by religious, educational, social, and recreational institutions.

"Nice girls don't let boys do that," was the mildest of warnings, followed by threats of dire punishment for seductive behavior. Virginity, chastity, abstinence from sexual foreplay beyond kissing were the ideals of virtue. Rare were the parents and counselors who would inform young women of available birth-control methods, for fear that such knowledge would lead to "loose" behavior.

Young men and adolescent boys too were, and are, taught sexual abstinence. "Save your seminal fluid." "You wouldn't want to marry a woman who isn't a virgin." "Don't let a loose woman lead you astray." "Don't get a girl with child." "Be clean in body and mind." These are values still taught by parents, religious institutions, schools, and such recreational institutions as Scouts and summer camps. But note that the greater burden of suspicion is put on the female.

Medical: Fear of Sexually Transmitted Diseases (STD). Until the availability of antibiotics in the 1940s, epidemics of gonorrhea and syphilis, then the most common of sexually transmitted diseases (also known as **venereal diseases** or **VD**), caused **sterility** (inability to reproduce) and life-threatening disability if not treated by prolonged and unpleasant medication. Since sexual intercourse with strangers or with more than one partner (**promiscuity**) greatly increases the risk of contracting sexually transmitted diseases, here, too, was a persuasive argument for sexual restraint---and still is.

I will have more to say later about sexually transmitted diseases, especially including chlamydia, herpes, and AIDS.

Respect and Love. Beyond these stern religious, sociological, and medical fears, a humane, informed, philosophical, and loving approach to sexual relations has always taught, and continues to teach, restraint. Parents, teachers, and religious leaders who have adopted this approach, based on reasoning rather than fear, believed---and believe---that children brought up to be considerate and respectful of their fellow human beings in all *other* circumstances will be *similarly* considerate and respectful in their *sexual* relations.

By example and by giving informed and respectful answers to questions, these adults fostered---and foster---strength of character through *moderation*, *patience*, and *endurance*, preaching that pleasure postponed until it can be responsibly, respectfully, and lovingly given and accepted is better than that given or taken for instant gratification.

These people also believed, and believe, that human beings need, from infancy through adolescence, the loving care of parents or some other family-like structure that will provide protection and guidance during the formative years. Standards and values instilled in the maturing child, by example and by reasoning, would, and will, inspire a sense of responsibility toward others---an understanding that responsible, considerate, trustworthy behavior is beneficial to society and oneself; an understanding that irresponsible, inconsiderate behavior is harmful to society and oneself.

Summary. These restraints are still with us. To a remarkable degree these pressures did restrain and continue to restrain the sexual impulsiveness of youths.

The Sexual Revolution

Differing social messages and pressures are always with us, however; and today are powerfully insistent. They make decisions on sexual behavior neither simple nor easy.

In 1948 was published the first volume of a major research project on human sexual behavior. It was entitled *Sexual Behavior in the Human Male,* by Alfred C. Kinsey, a respected biologist. A few years later the second volume, *Sexual Behavior in the Human Female*, was published. Popularly known as the Kinsey Reports, these statistical analyses of sexual behavior in America made clear that regardless of restraints and regardless of marital status, adults and youths are, and will be, sexually active. They also made clear to the public at large what every married woman knew: when husbands and wives gave in to the pleasures of sexual intercourse, women ran the ever-present risk of repeated pregnancies and increasing burdens of child rearing---this despite the use of birth controls then available.

In 1955 Doctors Gregory Pincus and John Rock and graduate student Min Chueh Chang developed an oral birth-control pill. Tested and approved in 1960 by the Food and Drug Administration, this "Pill" was marketed to allow sexual intercourse without the consequence of pregnancy. "The Pill," as it is popularly known, affects the balance of hormones necessary for ovulation, the release of an egg from an ovary. It is a virtually failure-proof preventive of pregnancy, and it immediately became a liberating aid to family planning. But the Pill is not taken without some risk to the health of the woman or girl who takes it, so it requires advice and prescription by a physician, and it cannot be bought "over the counter." Moreover, its use requires periodic check-ups so that physician and user can be assured its hormonal effects are doing no harm.

The Pill, plus publication of the Kinsey Reports, created a revolution in sexual behavior in Western civilization, allowing people to indulge in the pleasures of sexual intercourse, whether or not they were married, without fear of pregnancy. As a people, we in Western civilization were sexually liberated by knowledge of human sexual behavior and by the Pill. But the ethical and moral consequences have been neither easy nor simple, even world wide.

Taking a Stand

Where do I stand amidst these choices? Whether through strict moral and religious code, or fear of disgrace or disease, or through philosophical teaching, parents and society have idealized sexual intercourse as an intimate rather than a casual act, an expression of genuine affection between two people who are so attracted to each other that in marriage they wish to share responsibly and maturely in this most intense of intimacies. Community ordinances and state and federal laws have discouraged violation of this belief; and theater, movies, radio, television, newspapers, magazines, and books, until the 1970s, rarely questioned the standard.

You will find me with that group that teaches restraint through concern, respect, trust, and love for one's fellow human beings. I believe our biological capacity for sexual pleasure is an evolutionary insurance for survival of our species. We should enjoy it for its gift of ecstatic pleasure as well as for the marvel of procreation. It involves such powerful sensations and emotions, however, that the sexual urge can be as destructive as it can be creative. We human beings, unlike so-called lower animals, have to learn its nature and how to control its insistence, so that as partners we can enjoy it in a loving, trusting, mutually respectful regard for each other and for the consequences of our actions. It is my hope that this book will encourage such a philosophical approach to prevail.

GUIDELINES TO SAFE AND RESPONSIBLE SEXUAL BEHAVIOR

This part of *Sex and Consequences* repeats some of what has gone before, and it can be looked at almost separately. It is intended to guide you in ways that recognize both the idealistic and the realistic. Indeed, in our journey through life, I believe we must include the realistic with the ideal and the idealistic with the real.

ABSTINENCE AND A CONTROVERSY IN SEX EDUCATION

To repeat, I described sexual intercourse "under ideal circumstances" as "the ultimate act of love and trust between husband and wife." Ideally and despite the casual sex portrayed in all the media of our culture, there are boys and girls and men and women who wait until they are married, or are united as legal partners before engaging in sexual intercourse. They are virgins until their life's partnership, confirmed by religious ritual and/or by law, gives them their personal freedom to consummate that partnership.

Until the sexual revolution of the 1950s, many a bride and groom made their wedding night their first mutual invitation to, and acceptance of, sexual intercourse. All the restraints I mentioned in pages 64-66 were operative in such a decision, and are operative today for couples who choose to remain virginal until officially united.

This means sexual **abstinence** (abstaining from sexual intercourse) until union is recognized by the customs of one's religion and/or laws. And sexual abstinence is---without argument---the safest and most responsible principle of sexual behavior for a person to adopt. Certainly it is the first and most principled guidance and advice to give.

Because abstinence is the obvious first advice to give in classes on sex education, and because there is fear that knowledge of sexual behavior leads to sexual activity, many publicly-funded sex education courses teach abstinence as the *only* behavior model. Parents, school boards, politicians, law makers, religious leaders, and health officials, however, find themselves in controversy over whether abstinence alone should be taught. Health problems are now becoming the most persuasive argument for broader sex education. The life-threatening pandemic (worldwide epidemic) of AIDS demands broader education, and there are other considerations too. The controversy requires open examination among young people and their parents and other adult counselors.

Let us examine and discuss the following questions: Is abstinence in *all* instances the most trusting, the most loving, and the most respectful attitude in a romantic relationship? Is abstinence *always* biologically and psychologically realistic? And how does it apply to homosexual relationships?

As romantic relationships develop into loving commitments, it is natural and appropriate that couples expect intimacies of each other. Getting to know one's romantic partner in a trusting and loving relationship makes human life truly wonderful. To refuse completely any sexual involvement in that relationship is to deny knowledge of a fundamental part of our human biological nature.

But the pathway to that knowledge is not without all kinds of temptations to go beyond what is wise and responsible. So I shall now discuss ideals and realities of sexual behavior other than abstinence, bearing in mind that abstinence remains a realistic ideal.

First Sexual Experience

By "first sexual experience" I mean a sexually stimulating experience significant enough that the person knows she or he has passed from childhood innocence into a new and unfolding knowledge of life and sex. I do not necessarily mean the ultimate act of sexual intercourse; rather, I mean an event or incident that produces an intense, never-before-felt sexual sensation. We---you and I and your parents---should hope that this first sexual experience would occur after you have passed from childhood into adolescence, and that it would happen in circumstances developing from natural curiosity and unforced discovery, when you are alone or in the loving and gentle company of someone of like age and innocence.

With girls, menarche is a profound physiological initiation into womanhood, but it differs from the arousal, or excitement, of sexual knowingness. This arousal may be short of orgasm, possibly through romantic and intimate closeness with that someone of like age and innocence, or it may be the experience of actual orgasm through such an intense and intimate closeness or through masturbatory stimulation. This first orgasm may feel so strange and intense as to seem almost painful.

With boys, the first experience is most likely orgasm and ejaculation through a wet dream or through masturbation, or through intense and intimate closeness with someone, one would hope, of like age and innocence. As with girls, this first orgasm may feel so strangely intense as to be almost painful.

As I stated, it is best that the first sexual experience develop naturally from self-discovery or mutually shared discovery based on responsible knowledge. With another person, it should not be "the expected thing to do" that our TV and commercial cultures imply. The social implications of the casual sexual behavior displayed on TV and in movies put a terrible burden of expectations on real-life people, with consequences that cannot be anticipated and which are rarely considered in these media. The intimacy of sexual activity between people demands mutual respect and affection and trust and self-control. And it demands knowledge of health consequences as well as social and psychological consequences.

AVOIDING SEXUAL PREDATORS

Too often the case histories of adults with sexual problems reveal first experiences that were traumatic and frightening. Whatever the first sexual experience may be, there are ways of avoiding trauma and fear--- and of preventing trauma and fear in others. Here are some precautions, some of which I have listed more briefly elsewhere.

Be wary of more experienced persons of either sex who are anxious to indoctrinate you or force you into some sexual act. Be discreet, and discreetly turn them down. Example: "I'm not sure what you're getting at, but you're making me uncomfortable. Please don't go on with this." In turn, never force anyone or entice an innocent person to share in a sexual experience or act of yours. Avoid indoctrinating others who are younger, less experienced, less mature than yourself. And never entice an adult.

Especially avoid sexual advances from adults. Heterosexual or homosexual, they usually begin with friendly conversation that too quickly gets into questions and suggestions about sexual attitudes and behavior, followed by hugging and inappropriate touching Such advances from adults of either sex, whether strangers or well known to you, are frightening and potentially dangerous. Most adult advances come from people one knows: an uncle or aunt, a neighbor, family friend, grandparent, even a parent, a brother or sister, a teacher, a priest, a coach. In such instances, firm, repeated refusal to cooperate is usually enough. If verbal and physical rejection don't produce immediate retreat, shouting for help is a quick alternative. But if the male (or female) predator is physically aggressive, self-protection, such as kicking or punching, even in the genital area, may be necessary to free oneself. Not, however, if the assailant is armed. Quick and loud reaction is the best defense. Of course, you must report such incidents. The law requires reporting to police, immediately if intercourse has occurred (followed by emergency contraception). And to nearest of kin whom you trust. You will be saving yourself and others from trauma by speaking up and speaking out against such abuses.

And, of course, avoid the advances of strangers. Children and youths of either sex are attractive to predators on the prowl in automobiles, trucks, and playgrounds, or lurking at public toilets, rock concerts, and on the Internet.

Internet Predators. Lying in wait to seduce the innocent, to inflame sex addicts, and to relieve the naive (and the corrupted, too) of their money, are the sex links on the Internet. The most innocent search can suddenly open up channels of pornography. When that happens, click it off immediately! Don't allow your curiosity to explore it! The sex merchants know exactly how to lure you into depraved views and then hook you. More insidious are the "chat rooms." In search of an Internet pal, you can establish what seems to you an innocent friendship with a stranger and unwittingly become the prey of someone entirely (and perhaps dangerously) different from your imagined correspondent. Real friends are those you can look in the eye, in person.

More about predators and forced acts is on pages 81-83, 97, 98. Now let's back off such threatening subject matter and resume realistic discussions while upholding ideals.

Shared Sexual Activities

If two or more people, through speech, visual stimulation, and/or physical contact, arouse sexual desire in each other, one could say that they are sharing in activity that can be interpreted as sexual. One would suppose that a friendly kiss or handhold doesn't count. But a lingering kiss or a caressing handhold indicates romantic feelings. These are harmless, generally accepted behavior, though frowned upon if too publicly displayed. Consider, however, the general heterosexual reaction to such affection displayed by same-sex couples and you have an example of how difficult it is for homosexuals to establish romantic relationships.

At what level of intensity does shared sexual activity become consequential enough to bring into play the array of personal and societal concerns that affect our conduct as responsible human beings?

Deep kissing, or French kissing, open-mouth kissing, is an intimacy that can easily be misunderstood. Because it is standard in romantic movies and TV dramas and TV mating contests, it would seem almost expected. It can be interpreted, however, as an invitation to foreplay (defined on page 38). Already caution is the watchword. For the couple so involved but with no intentions of going further, it is a fairly easy point from which to say, "No further." This assumes, however, that the sharing couple are in only each other's company. It assumes also that a responsible and caring adult, preferably a parent, is nearby and within hearing and calling distance. The intensity and temptations of shared sexual activity increase rapidly under the pressure of group situations at carelessly supervised parties, and they are dangerously fueled to recklessness by the introduction of alcohol and drugs.

Now when I refer to a sharing couple, I would hope---for reasons that will soon become clear---that the two people are emotionally mature enough to have developed a true understanding of each other. This means respecting and trusting each other. It means sharing interests and, most important, it means a commitment to share any sexual activity responsibly and only with each other. But as early as middle school, some young people knowing each other no better than first-time acquaintances by e-mail or at a party are exploring sexual activities far more intense than kissing and handholding. By this I mean touching and fondling breasts and each other's genitals, going on to mutual masturbation and mouth-to-genitals stimulation ("oral sex," which is often only for the gratification of the boy).

Promiscuity. Somehow such activities have acquired a reputation of being "not real sex" and "OK because they don't risk pregnancy." But such behavior is not only a violation of one's privacy and a reduction of one's sex to the level of instant gratification; it is an acceptance of **promiscuity**. Promiscuity, as defined earlier, means sexual activity with several or many partners without regard to lasting commitment.

Promiscuity is totally destructive of trustworthy relationships at any level. (Think about that. It's probably the strongest statement in this book, but it's true, isn't it?) It is also an immediate avenue to sexually transmitted diseases (STDs).

Self-Esteem and Promiscuity

Boys. When a boy feels he has to prove himself by demonstrating his sexual prowess, he is reducing his personality to the level of his genitals. Sadly, this too is an attitude promoted by our commercial society. Male models for underwear, beachwear, teen magazines, body building, and beer ads display bulked-up muscles and torsos bared almost to the pubic level---all suggesting that genitals are the prize. Certainly the masturbatory gestures by males on MTV and similar entertainment blatantly promote sexual prowess. And focus on genitals is the primary emphasis of the pornography industry. What is there of lasting interest and attraction in such displays and activities? Nothing for the mind, nothing to encourage understanding, caring, respect, intellectual bonding, which are the qualities of personality and character on which true friendship and love are based. Commercially, sexual activity is prized only for brief conquest and gratification---nothing more. This may seem Darwinian in promoting reproduction, but it is contrary to the preservation of our species: By denying our intellectual capacity for civilized conversation, love, and nurturing, we deny the family values essential to the healthy breeding of generations. By reducing sexual intimacy to the level of temporary thrills or bathroom vulgarity, a boy lowers his self-esteem to that same level, and---even worse---he lowers his esteem for his sexual partner to that of a receptacle.

Girls. When a girl feels that sexual attractiveness is the only key to her social success, she is reducing her personality to breasts, buttocks, and genitals. This too is promoted by our commercial society. Underwear, beachwear, and social wear worn by female models in magazines, TV ads, and TV entertainments direct attention immediately to these body parts as though they are all a young woman needs to be popular. And the girls and young women who model such apparel have dieted to skeletal thinness while bulking their breasts and lips with silicone gels. Pelvic thrusts and mouth-and-tongue gestures in sex comedies, MTV, and similar entertainment blatantly invite sexual penetration. Sexual attractiveness for just the few moments of a boy's orgasm, or hers, denies all the lasting pleasures and bonds of conversation, mutual understanding, and the mutual care and trust and respect between two civilized and intelligent human beings. Preservation of the human species involves *lasting pleasures and bonds* to provide us with the patience and endurance to ensure the nurturing care of the next generations. By making herself only the object of a boy's mindless urge for his own sexual gratification, a girl lowers her self-esteem to that of a receptacle, and she does nothing for the boy's character development.

I have more to say about promiscuity, this time in relation to sexually transmitted diseases, but first some more advice about irresponsible and responsible sexual behavior.

Taking Responsibility
And Acquiring Wisdom
In Shared Sexual Behavior

An ideal for shared sexual activity is the mutual sharing between two married or legally committed adults, faithful, loving, responsible, respectful, understanding, informed, and trusting. For heterosexuals the consequences of such shared sexual activity are a lasting life of loving companionship and the strengthening of the bonds of marriage toward procreation and parenting. For homosexuals, through mutual understanding and respect, the two partners can freely explore, physically and in conversation, the pleasures of shared sexual activity as part of their loving, lasting commitment to each other. Ideally, such shared sexual activity can be playful, romantic, intense, relaxed---directed toward bringing a baby to the union, or joyfully indulged in solely for pleasure, or both. There is nothing cheap or demeaning or furtive about it. Obviously, this definition is of people who have matured beyond puberty and adolescence. My principal concern here is for young people who---outside the supervision of caring and responsible adults---may be overwhelmed by love and sexual desire. I would be irresponsible if I didn't recognize that some youths are not going to *abstain* from sexual activity. For this reason I shall be explicit about the sexual activities that you, as young readers, hear about and see and will be tempted to try. And I shall be explicit about the consequences of these activities

CONSEQUENCES OF YOUNG PEOPLE'S SHARED SEXUAL ACTIVITIES

Whether or not you choose abstinence, you have heard or will be hearing and reading in the media about a variety of sexual activities that some of your peers are indulging in, casually or for thrills or for genuine affection. You should know the consequences of these activities. First I shall discuss shared sexual activities, exclusive of vaginal intercourse, that induce orgasm. Then I shall discuss vaginal intercourse and its consequences. By discussing these activities, however, I do not mean to create the impression of recommendation. What a loving married couple may do in the privacy of the bedroom has consequences quite different from the consequences of the same activities indulged in by young unmarried people. Among young people shared activities directed only toward orgasm make sexual union commonplace. They blur the difference between lust and love, and they can make the later sexual commitment of marriage seem less valuable. Since sexually transmitted diseases (STDs) must also be considered, I shall mention STDs briefly here and at more length later. Bear in mind, therefore, that this is about your future as well as your present.

Shared Sexual Activities Exclusive of Vaginal Intercourse

Mutual masturbation, heterosexual or homosexual, is the least risky of shared activities that can induce orgasm. Gently practiced, it gives reciprocal pleasure that can be stopped short of orgasm. Free of STDs it is a safe and pleasurable alternative to abstinence or promiscuity. But if either partner is, or has been, promiscuous, STDs are a risk. Contact of hands with genitals and semen provides the possibility of STDs if promiscuity has been involved (or if either partner has been infected with HIV, the AIDS virus, through drug use). Therefore, partners in mutual masturbation, heterosexual or homosexual, must be totally honest and frank about each other's past sexual activities. To ensure safety from STD when partners have any reason to doubt each other, a male should wear a condom (see pages 86-87), and partners' hands should be free of abrasions.

Oral sex (see also "hooking up") is riskier than mutual masturbation. Oral contact with genitals, semen, vaginal secretions, and blood makes it risky, especially if there are cuts or abrasions in or on one's mouth or genitals. Popular opinion may lead you to think otherwise, but a partner infected with the AIDS virus and/or the herpes virus can transmit the virus through oral/genital contact. Since promiscuous sexual behavior is likely to expose a person unknowingly to infection with STDs, people practicing oral sex are at risk unless both partners have been scrupulously true only to each other and neither has been infected. Without such complete honesty in this relationship, a male must wear a condom when being orally stimulated and should avoid direct oral contact with the naked genitalia of his partner. This same scrupulous attention to safe health procedure must apply to homosexual as well as heterosexual partners.

The riskiest, most hazardous sexual behavior is anal sex, also known as sodomy (a legal term also applied to oral sex). Among heterosexual partners it is sometimes a substitute for vaginal intercourse and an avoidance of pregnancy. Among homosexual males it tends to be an expected practice. Penetration of anus and rectum is exceptionally hazardous to anal muscles and to the delicate tissues of the rectum. These easily torn tissues can become infected, and in females proximity of rectal tissues to vaginal tissues increases this hazard. Even when such precautions as an enema and sterile lubrication are used (and they should be), risk is high for damage and infection. Moreover, anal intercourse is a primary source for transmission of HIV and hepatitis B, both of which are associated with promiscuity among heterosexuals as well as homosexuals. Indeed, it is among male homosexuals practicing anal intercourse that AIDS was first diagnosed in the early 1980s. The likely mixture of blood and semen between partners in anal intercourse can have deadly consequences. It is imperative, therefore, that any male (heterosexual or homosexual) penetrating the anus of his partner wear a condom externally lubricated with a sterile, water-soluble gel. This means every time and under all circumstances.

A final consideration of consequences of anal intercourse is the pain of penetration. Assuming mutual consent of the partners, what is the cost in personal dignity, mutual respect, and caring love?

I'm sorry to have to be so frank about these matters, but when you and your peers are exposed to such behavior through friends, news media, pornography, and elsewhere, I am obligated to discuss consequences and responsibilities. Among the emotional and social consequences of such intense sexual activities can be loss of self-esteem and reputation. Boys and girls boast and gossip about their sexual exploits, whisper about reputations of other girls and boys, scribble such messages on desk tops and bathroom walls, and, devastatingly nowadays, broadcast pictures and slander via e-mail. So just as you would not want your own reputation ruined, you must keep silent among peers about your own behavior and the behavior of others. It is far better, of course, to avoid such intense sexual activity. Thus you can see why abstinence is a realistic virtue.

WHAT TO DO WHEN YOU THINK SHARED SEXUAL ACTIVITY BEGINS TO GET TOO INTENSE

Here is some advice on how to extricate yourself from situations in which you believe sexual activity is getting too intense or is leading to promiscuous behavior. And here you have to take responsibility for yourself, regardless of what is popular or supposedly expected in a "go with the flow" society

The most respectful approach is simply to say, "I think we've gone far enough. Let's cool off. We oughtn't to get so intimate." A respectful couple, alone, can easily do this, but there are those times when the more aggressive partner, usually the boy, puts up an argument. A standard argument is something like this: "I have an erection. It hurts. It's bad for me. You have to let me do it." A candid response is, "Relax.

It's not bad for you. I'm not going to let you. Go read a magazine till it dies down. Then we'll behave ourselves." If that doesn't suffice, and you worry he might become physically aggressive, try a little sarcasm: "Take it into the bathroom and don't come back until you've done what you had to." If the girl is the aggressor and she ridicules the boy's manliness with such questions as, "What's the matter? Scared? Don't you like girls?" His response might be, "No, I'm not scared. Are you scared I might not like you unless you put out?"

In a group, it's more difficult to stand against peer pressure; but you might be surprised to discover what the courage of strong resistance can do to quickly lower erotic fever all around: "Oh come on, everyone. This is ridiculous. We're all acting like a bunch of horny cats and dogs. Turn up the lights. Let's go somewhere and get something to eat." Usually a girl is the more courageous, but a boy can be just as persuasive.

Sexual Assault and Rape. A clear danger in sexually heated circumstances is **sexual assault**, in which a boy becomes so aggressive that, against a girl's expressed refusal, he threatens her and forcefully fondles her breasts and genitals. When a girl senses coming danger, she can usually stop it by *shouting* "No!" Sexual assault is frightening, illegal, and severely punishable by law. Going beyond sexual assault, if the boy verbally and/or physically forces the girl to yield to sexual intercourse or sodomy, including oral sex, he is guilty of **rape**. Rape is a violent and terrifying act and, threatened or committed, it is illegal and severely punishable by law. If it seems imminent, the girl must not be immobilized by fear. She should not hesitate to cry out and to get out of reach. This will usually deter the boy. (More about predatory sexual behavior on pages 73-74, 97, 98.)

Drugs and alcohol are fuels for assault and rape. Under their influence boys and girls lose self-control, and girls become especially vulnerable to physical assault. Good reason to avoid substance abuse! And in sobriety girls and boys should be aware of danger signals. Boys who are tempted to bully and control and are excessively demanding of sexual gratification, should be so concerned about their own aggressiveness that they should seek counseling to modify these tendencies. And parents should express, and act on, their concerns about a son's behavior patterns that might lead to abusiveness, sexual or otherwise. Parents can readily size up a son's inappropriate behavior in social situations and must not close their eyes to it. The subject of rape is so important that parents and school counselors should educate themselves and their offspring and students on how to avoid forced sexual acts and how to respond if they occur, including early access to emergency contraception (see page 84).

Among homosexual couples, male or female, the same techniques can be used to reduce intensity of sexual excitement and activity. Boys are as likely as girls to be in situations where an aggressive male can be frightening and dangerous. When a boy, homosexual or heterosexual, is in a situation where a bully (boy or man) starts to "come on" to him, he'd better be prepared not only to say, "That's not for me," and be aggressively firm but also have a way to escape. One of the male homosexual stereotypes is the very masculine, bullying kind. If by chance or adventure, a boy is ganged up on by several such males, or even one, he'd better extricate himself quickly, lest he be raped. Unsupervised locker rooms and public men's lavatories are places where aggressive male homosexual behavior can take place and where a boy, heterosexual or homosexual, can be ganged up on if he is alone.

What to Do When Sexual Activity Leads to Vaginal Intercourse

Contraception

For sexually active heterosexual couples, pregnancy is always a possible consequence. A child should not be brought into this world unless it can be lovingly cared for by adults emotionally mature enough and financially responsible enough to see to its sustained rearing and education. Until these conditions are a reality, the couple should rigorously avoid conception. **Contraception** (conception prevention), though forbidden by some religions, is the obvious choice for couples who insist on the pleasure of intercourse without the consequence of pregnancy.

If instead of abstinence a girl has chosen to be sexually active, she should confide with responsible adults, her parents preferably, especially if she has a good, confidential relationship with one or both. A trusted family doctor would be another choice. So also a trusted school counselor, a religious counselor. It is vital that she be effectively informed and counseled about the consequences to her well-being, to her reputation, and to the rest of her life. She should certainly know also about the availability and effectiveness of the most commonly used contraceptives. And let us hope that any involved male brings himself, or is brought, to similar counseling---for the same reasons.

Biochemical Contraception

The Birth Control Pill. "The Pill" (see page 68) is by far the most effective contraceptive, but not a protection against STDs. The Pill is for females, not males, so the burden of responsibility is on girls and women. Moreover, it must be prescribed and overseen by a physician because it affects the hormones related to reproduction, and for a few girls and women the Pill's hormonal consequences can be very harmful to health.

The Emergency Contraception ("EC") Pill. Another contraceptive pill, also affecting reproductive hormonal balance, has become useful as a "morning-after" method of preventing ovulation or preventing uterine implantation of the fertilized egg. The "emergency contraception pill," commonly referred to as "the EC," is for such unprotected sex emergencies as a broken condom (see page 87) or reckless or forced sexual encounter. To be effective it must be taken within 72 hours after intercourse, preferably 48 hours. Because it is expensive ($30-$40 per dose), may cause nausea, and interferes with the menstrual cycle, it is not to be used casually or regularly as a birth control. Produced under the name "Plan B," it is currently available without prescription to women 18 or older, and it is not a protection against STDs. Note that the responsibility is placed on the girl or woman, not the male.

The Contraceptive Patch. "The Patch," like a square band-aid, can be applied to various parts of the female body. Its contraceptive hormones are absorbed through the skin, and they affect hormonal balance in such a way as to prevent ovulation and to prevent sperms from entering the uterus. Use of The Patch requires careful adherence to directions, including exact renewal of application every week. It is *not* an *emergency* contraceptive; it *does* require medical prescription. It is not a protection against STDs.

Contraception by Injection. Depo Provera is a hormonal contraceptive intended to be administered to women only by health care providers. Injected every 13 weeks, it prevents pregnancy by suppressing ovulation. As with other biochemical contraceptives, its effects must be monitored, and it must be administered with careful adherence to directions. It is not a protection against STDs.

Effective as these biochemical contraceptives are against impregnation, none should be used without prior knowledge and/or medical or clinical supervision.

Barrier Contraception

Less expensive, less effective contraceptives are *physical barriers* between sperm and egg. The three most common are the **spermicidal sponge**, the **diaphragm**, and the **condom**. *The condom is the only one that protects against sexually transmitted diseases.*

The Spermicidal Sponge. The spermicidal sponge is disk shaped, with a concave surface that fits the cervix. It is made of polyurethane treated with a spermicide (sperm killer). Spermicidal sponges can be purchased without prescription in drugstores. Before insertion they must be made wet (to activate the spermicide). Practice is required for insertion and removal. The folded sponge is inserted in the vagina and placed over the cervix. Removal after intercourse involves an attached ribbon loop. Spermicidal sponges are about 80 percent effective as contraceptives, but only if properly inserted a few minutes (or as long as 24 hours) before intercourse, and kept in place six hours after intercourse. *They are not a protection against sexually transmitted diseases.*

The Diaphragm. The diaphragm, about 80 percent effective, is a circular rubber cap that fits over the cervix. In its rim a metal spring keeps it in place once it is inserted. Disadvantages are that it requires a prescription and special fitting inside the vagina and over the cervix. Moreover, the wearer must smear it with spermicidal jelly before inserting it. Insertion should be no less than an hour before intercourse, and removal no less than six hours after intercourse. Its insertion prior to intercourse is unpleasant, its removal after intercourse is messy, and it is no barrier to disease and infection.

The Condom. The condom is now the recommended contraceptive. It is not only a male-worn barrier against conception but also a protection against *infection from* and *spread of* sexually transmitted diseases (see also pages 97-98 for homosexual use of condoms). Since it can be subject, however, to failures if its wearing is not understood, the following explanations are vital to its safe and effective use.

A condom is a thin latex sheath that fits snugly over the entire length of the erect penis. Condoms are inexpensive and available in any drugstore, where they are sold in small boxes containing several. They are also available free in college infirmaries, in some high-school infirmaries, and in family-counseling agencies. Each condom is rolled up and sealed, usually with a water-soluble lubricating gel, in a sterile package. At a condom's end may be a tip that serves to hold ejaculated semen. Regardless of such a tip, the most important precaution in putting on a condom is first to pinch its end to ensure adequate space for semen. Then, holding the pinched end against the head of the erect penis, unroll the condom over the entire shaft of the penis. (Pull back the foreskin of an uncircumcised penis before unrolling the condom.)

Immediately after ejaculation, to prevent the condom from slipping off and spilling semen, the wearer should hold onto its base as he withdraws his penis. And caring of his partner, he will have figured out how to dispose of the condom and clean himself.

Objections to a condom are several: To put it on interferes with spontaneity of romantic love making, and to wear it reduces somewhat the male's pleasurable sensation of intercourse. However, users learn to make putting on the condom a pleasurable part of foreplay, and the reduced sensitivity can prolong the pleasure of intercourse. Another objection is that condoms are not always failure-proof contraceptives or fail-safe preventives of STD. The following fail-safe precautions will greatly reduce the possibility of a condom tearing during intercourse: Condoms should be obtained from a reliable drugstore or other dispensary, and because of short shelf life, their date of manufacture is important to know. Condoms should not be kept where overheating (as in an automobile glove compartment) and pressure (as in a sat-upon wallet) can affect their resilience. And if lubrication is desired, it should be with a water-soluble gel, never an oil- or petroleum-based lubricant. These simple observances make the condom the safest and most reliable of barrier contraceptives.

Condoms are not only the most easily available contraceptives and best disease preventives; their use puts on both male *and* female an easy responsibility to avoid pregnancy and disease. Anyone---male or female---avoiding pregnancy but likely to engage in sexual intercourse, should be prepared by having purchased condoms, and the girl or woman should *insist* that her male partner wear one during sexual intercourse. Parents should suppress embarrassment about discussing with their sons and daughters the use and importance of condoms.

Which gets me back to the admonition, however, that abstinence until marriage makes life sexually safe and simpler for young people and adults.

Inadequate Methods of Avoiding Pregnancy When Having Vaginal Intercourse

The following methods are neither safe nor effective in contraception or in disease prevention.

Rhythm. The so-called rhythm or "cycle-based" or "fertility awareness" method is based on awareness of the woman's most likely fertile time between menstrual periods. Supposedly by avoiding intercourse during the variable ten days when ovulation may be occurring, the young woman is "safe" from pregnancy. Because of the irregular nature of the menstrual cycle, however, even among women whose periods seem predictable, the rhythm method is like playing Russian roulette.

Withdrawal. Withdrawal of the penis before ejaculation is an even less effective way of avoiding pregnancy. It requires an acute sense of timing and more self-control than most couples have during the intensity of approaching orgasm. Moreover, there is likelihood that spermatozoa are in the male's pre-ejaculatory secretions.

The Douche. The douche, an attempt to wash out or irrigate the vagina after intercourse, is a really foolish method. Based on ignorance but often spoken of with misleading authority, the introduction of carbonated or plain water into the vagina as a douche after intercourse is not only hygienically dangerous but certainly ineffective.

Beware of peer advice on contraception or any other such advice that cannot be verified by medical authority. Again, abstinence is the simple, safe alternative to the temptations and consequences of shared sexual activity.

Pregnancy

I must here reiterate to pre-adolescent and adolescent readers that you are not ready for the responsibility of motherhood or fatherhood and the long-term love and care and expense that go with being a parent. As an adolescent you are physically mature enough to reproduce, but your emotional, social, and intellectual developments, which are uneven at best, need some years to catch up. Young and inexperienced psyches aren't ready for the consequences of fully gratifying the powerful sexual urges that commercial and entertainment industries imply can be gratified without consequences. This is why I devote so much space and thought to consequences and responsibilities if you do experiment with shared sexual activities.

What if premarital adolescent sexual activity leads to pregnancy? What should the young couple do? I would hope, as the first response, the girl would be able to tell her parents. Of all situations requiring loving and responsible parents, this is probably the most crucial. And I would hope that the involved boy would be able to speak to his parents and that the two families could get together to work out their responsibilities.

To parents and children reading this book, I urge that you maintain the courage and love that enable you to talk with each other about such emotion-laden topics. Dealing with unwanted pregnancy is difficult, emotionally painful, and morally consequential. Whether to allow the embryo to develop into an infant that will be lovingly and responsibly cared for or to terminate the pregnancy by abortion is a decision fraught with personal, religious, ethical, and societal consequences. Though opponents of abortion denigrate Planned Parenthood, it is an agency that will inform you (with parents, one would hope, but without them if necessary) about procedures for carrying pregnancy to birth and responsible rearing, or for terminating the pregnancy. Knowing these choices, seek the advice of the wisest, most responsible, confidential, and caring adult, or adults, you know; and this would include your family physician as well as your parents and a religious counselor.

Sexually Transmitted Diseases

We human beings are in constant battle against all kinds of diseases, the transmission of some of which we have little control over. We do, however, have some control over STDs. STDs are also known as STIs, or sexually transmitted infections. They were once known as VDs, or venereal diseases (venereal referring to the Roman goddess of love, Venus). Here I shall discuss explicitly the consequences and responsibilities related to sexual activities and the most common STDs. **But before I proceed, I must stress use of the condom as the best preventive of STDs, *short of abstinence*; so reread the passage on condom use (pages 86-87).**

Chlamydial and Plasmal Diseases. The most common STDs are chlamydial and plasmal. Chlamydial disease is caused by a microscopic parasite, *Chlamydia trachomatis*, easily transmitted by an infected male or female. In girls and women symptoms from infection through vaginal intercourse may be any or all of the following: yellowish vaginal discharge, frequent and painful urination, painful vaginal intercourse, and pain in the pelvic (low abdominal) region. Infection from oral sex is likely to cause a sore throat. Infection from anal sex is likely to cause inflammation of the anus and rectum. Chlamydial disease can fool girls and women, however, because it may be symptomless for considerable time after infection.

In boys and men, symptoms appear within a week to month after intercourse with an infected partner. Mild urethral pain is followed by clear or mucous discharge. During one's sleep the mouth of the penis may be temporarily stuck closed by this discharge, which can stain underwear and bed clothes. Urination may be painful. Infection from oral sex with an infected male or female partner will cause a sore throat. Infection from anal penetration by an infected partner will cause inflammation of the anus and rectum.

Untreated, chlamydial infection may become symptom free after a few weeks, but in girls and women it will then cause inflammation of the oviducts, which (again, if untreated) can result in death. In boys and men, untreated chlamydial infection will cause narrowing of the urethra and permanent inflammation damage to the epididymis, resulting in sterility (inability to produce spermatozoa and have children). New and more virulent chlamydia bacteria have recently been found in a few infected homosexual and bisexual men. All the more reason to avoid risky sexual activity.

Plasmal diseases are similar in infectiousness and symptoms. Fortunately, chlamydial and plasmal diseases can readily be cured by specific antibiotics if caught in time. Since they are such common STDs, anyone the least suspicious of infection after sexual activity should see a reputable doctor. Some schools and colleges now offer free and easy examinations for detection of these STDs.

Chlamydial and plasmal infections are easily and unknowingly transmitted through **promiscuous** sexual activity. A reason for condom use or abstinence.

Genital Warts and Cervical Cancer. A common STD is genital warts, also known as **HPV** (human papilloma virus). Genital warts are unlike warts that sometimes develop on hands. In infected girls and women, they grow on the vulva, on skin between vulva and anus, and in the vagina and on the cervix. At first small, moist, pink pimples, they rapidly grow into cauliflower-like clusters. In infected boys and men, genital warts may first appear just behind the head of the penis, especially the undersurface, also in the mouth of the penis and on the shaft. Among infected people practicing anal intercourse, they are likely to be found around the anus and in the rectum. Bare skin contact with infected bare skin **unprotected by condom** is a source of transmission. Since genital warts take 1 to 6 months to appear after infection, the disease can be transmitted unknowingly. Minor surgery and local applications of medicines are usually effective in early stages, but there is no sure cure for genital warts (antibiotics don't work on viruses).

Cervical-cancer-causing strains of HPV are becoming more common than they were only a few years ago, and are now being detected among sexually active teenagers. Vaccines have been developed to **prevent** such HPV infection but **must** be taken by a girl **before** exposure, not after; thus **before a girl becomes sexually active**. A caring relationship between parents and children is therefore vital to open, frank discussion of disease prevention and possible lifelong HPV consequences to a sexually active teenager.

Genital Herpes. Another common STD is genital herpes (HERPeez), also known as **HSV**, or herpes simplex virus Type 2. It does not respond to antibiotics, and no vaccine has yet been developed to prevent infection. Therefore the saying, "Herpes is forever." Symptoms appear within a few days of contact of naked genitals with the naked genitals of an infected partner. They are painful, itchy sores that ulcerate, become crusty, then disappear within two weeks but leave scars. These symptoms periodically reappear and disappear and are most infectious when they reappear. In infected girls and women, they are most often found on the clitoris, the lips of the vulva, and the skin between vulva and anus. They may progress into the vagina and onto the cervix. In infected boys and men, the sores appear on the head of the penis and on the foreskin and shaft. In infected females and males involved in anal sex, the sores may appear around the anus and in the rectum. Oral sex with an infected partner can produce herpes sores in the mouth. Women infected with HSV are in danger of infecting their infants during childbirth.

"Fever blisters" or "cold sores," caused by herpes simplex virus Type 1, though not labeled STD, can also infect male or female genitals through oral sex, even if genitals are washed with soap and water immediately afterwards.

Transmission of HSV can occur by skin contact with herpes-infected skin **not covered by a condom**. Though there is no known cure for genital herpes, people who suspect infection should see a reputable doctor for diagnosis, treatment, and advice.

Gonorrhea. Historically-known STDs are gonorrhea (gahnoREEah) and syphilis. Both are highly infectious and have been the sources of STD epidemics throughout history. They were the most common VDs (venereal diseases) of World Wars I and II among sexually active partners **unprotected by condoms**. Infection with gonorrhea (also known as "the clap") is evident in males within a few days of sexual contact with an infected partner. In infected girls and women there may be pain in urination and maybe vaginal discharge, but usually no symptoms until the disease is well settled in. Thus infected girls and women can transmit it unknowingly. First symptoms in infected boys and men are mild pain in the urethra, then pain during urination, followed by discharge of pus. The pus is highly infectious, so the infected person should immediately report the symptoms and be isolated. Other symptoms are redness and swelling at the mouth of the penis. Among infected partners who practice **promiscuous**, **unprotected** oral sex and anal sex, gonorrhea will infect mouth and throat, anus and rectum.

Gonorrhea is easily treated with antibiotics, since it is a bacterial infection, but if left untreated, it will spread to the epididymis and vas deferens in males and to the oviducts in females, damaging these organs and causing sterility (inability to reproduce).

Because of the danger of gonorrhea becoming epidemic, anyone suspecting infection in himself or herself should immediately seek medical attention and identify anyone with whom he or she has had sexual contact. This is a vital responsibility, and it is why it is so important for young people and their parents to be able to speak frankly with each other.

Syphilis. Syphilis (also known as lues and "the pox" or "the great pox") has been an epidemic STD from time to time over centuries, and descriptions of its ravages appear in literature and medical texts dating back to the Renaissance and earlier. It is caused by a microscopic, spiral organism called a **spirochete** (SPYrokeet). A spirochete-infected person can infect others through sexual activity or through contaminated needles in drug use. Entrance of sexually induced spirochetes is through infectious contact with skin abrasions and such mucous membranes as in the mouth, vagina, and rectum. Heavy kissing, oral-genital contact, and anal and vaginal intercourse with an infected person are certain to produce infection. The spirochetes thrive in the blood stream and rapidly move to other organs, including the central nervous system, but outside the body they are short lived. The first obvious symptom of syphilis appears at the spirochetes' point of entrance. It looks like a reddish skin eruption. Painlessly this eruption ulcerates and forms a hard base which, if scratched, produces pus rather than blood. It is called a **chancre** (pronounced SHANKer). In infected girls and women, the chancre most often appears on the vulva or the cervix or the area between the vulva and the anus. In infected boys and men, it usually appears on the penis, but anal sex from an infected partner will result in anal and rectal chancres. Syphilis is becoming more and more common among homosexuals. Oral sex, even deep kissing, with an infected partner, male or female, heterosexual or homosexual, can produce a chancre on lips, tongue, mouth, throat. Chancres can also appear on hands or any other part of the body where spirochetes enter through a break in the skin.

The earliest stage of syphilis is called **primary syphilis**. If the infected person is untreated, the chancre will disappear and the person may seem free of disease. But within several months a rash (hence the old-fashioned name "pox") will break out. This is the symptom of **secondary syphilis**. This too will disappear. If untreated, secondary syphilis will develop into **tertiary syphilis**, often years later. Untreated tertiary syphilis affects the heart and the nervous system and is fatal.

Like gonorrhea, syphilis is so infectious that anyone suspicious of symptoms should immediately see a physician and be prepared to give a specific account of any and all people with whom one has been in sexual contact over the preceding three months. This is a moral responsibility. Do you see why **promiscuity** is so risky and irresponsible?

The good news is that early stages of syphilis are easily cured with antibiotics. The bad news is that promiscuous behavior can result in reinfection. Again, you must surely see the arguments in favor of **abstinence**, **fidelity**, and **condom use**.

Hepatitis B (HBV). Hepatitis B is a viral liver infection transmitted not only through sexual activity but also through illicit drug injection with used needles. Other sources of infection are eating carelessly-prepared, raw shellfish; contact with feces (FEESeez, bowel movement) from infected people (including contact with unwashed hands in neglected public washrooms); and exposure to infected blood. Person-to-person transmission is often unwitting since the disease is most infectious in its earliest stages, before symptoms appear. As a sexually transmitted disease, it is more often detected among homosexual boys and men than among heterosexuals. This is often because of contamination with infected fecal (FEEKel) matter from anal intercourse.

Symptoms of hepatitis B appear one to six weeks after infection. Loss of appetite, nausea, sometimes followed by hives and painful joints. Then dark urine. The clearest sign is yellowness in the whites of eyes and even the skin, a symptom known as **jaundice**. Anyone with these symptoms should immediately see a physician and avoid physical contact with others (as protection against transmitting the infection) until assured of no longer being infectious. If untreated, the patient runs the risk of permanent damage to the liver, in rare cases life-threatening damage, though some patients recover without incident.

Because HBV is a viral disease, antibiotics are useless in fighting it, so physician-regulated care is essential to recovery. Alcohol and illicit drugs can be life threatening during the illness.

Do you see the consequences of **promiscuity**? Do you see why many sex educators promote abstinence, and why, in addition, I urge fidelity and knowledge of condom use?

Yeast Infections. Yeast infections are usually *not* transmitted sexually. In women, however, they are not uncommon. Yeast is commonly present in the intestinal tract and on normal skin. Menstruation, dependence on antibiotics, and use of oral contraceptives tend to increase susceptibility to yeast infections. Symptoms are inflamed vulva and cheesy accumulations on the vaginal wall, accompanied by vaginal discharge. Also bladder pain and infection. In men there may be no symptoms, or there may be some discharge from the penis and inflammatory accumulation of cheesy substance under the foreskin. Men and women can unwittingly infect each other if one or the other is infected. Fortunately, yeast infections can be treated with specific antibiotics, and men can avoid infection---or if infected, their transmission of infection---by condom use.

AIDS

The diseases above are the more common STDs. There are others less common, but the STD getting most publicity and creating a worldwide scare is **AIDS**, the acronym for **a̱cquired i̱mmunod̲eficiency s̲yndrome**, caused by **HIV**, the **h̲uman i̱mmunodeficiency v̲irus** (technically a *retro*virus, which affects DNA in cells of the person infected).

AIDS is just what the full name implies; it is a complex of diseases developing in an infected person as a consequence of a breakdown of the wonderful immune system that normally protects us from all kinds of infections. Because antibiotics do not work against viruses, and because no vaccine has yet been developed to combat HIV, the eventual complex of diseases will kill the AIDS patient. There *are* expensive medicines that suppress and delay indefinitely the development of this sickness. Even so, HIV mutates readily into new varieties.

The illnesses that develop in full-blown AIDS include fever, general sick feeling, pneumonia, anemia, diarrhea, a cancer known as Kaposi's sarcoma (which first appears as purple blotches on the skin), and finally a dreadful wasting away. Because AIDS may not develop in an HIV-infected person until many months or even years after infection, anyone involved in risky sexual behavior can unwittingly transmit the virus and should be tested frequently and routinely for HIV infection. (Clinics will perform such tests while maintaining privacy, and now some schools and most colleges and universities will readily perform them. The tests are simple and quick, the results quickly available.)

AIDS was first described and diagnosed in the early 1980s among a few homosexual men who were dying of a mysterious wasting disease. When HIV was first isolated, it was found in the blood and semen of infected male homosexuals. Later, when women were found infected, HIV was discovered in their vaginal secretions as well as in their blood. It is also in breast milk of infected mothers and can thus be passed on to infants. **HIV is transmitted by commingling of any or all of these "bodily fluids" (including, to a lesser extent, saliva) between an uninfected and an HIV-infected person.** It is now found among men, women, youths, and children. Note, however, that HIV is not found in sweat and tears. **Primarily a sexually transmitted disease, it is also transmitted by infected people who take and give drugs by means of used needles and syringes.** Moreover, people infected with **gonorrhea** and/or **syphilis** are especially susceptible to infection with HIV. HIV and AIDS have spread worldwide, and millions of infected people are dying of AIDS.

Now I shall discuss what to fear and not to fear about transmission of HIV. First, what to fear, and how to avoid infection.

1. Beware of sexual contact with anyone sexually **promiscuous**. Such people, young or older, have probably had sexual union with someone infected with HIV. Abstinence, of course, is the surest way of avoiding infection. Use of condoms the next surest.

2. Beware of sexual activity with anyone whose sexual history is unknown to you. Even if that person seems trustworthy and claims to be HIV free, you risk infection if you indulge in sex play that results in mingling of bodily fluids.

3. Avoid parties at which sex, alcohol, and/or drugs are part of the scene. Such parties quickly fuel **promiscuity** and put every guest at risk, not only for STDs but also for rape and unwanted pregnancy.

4. Never inject drugs with used needles and/or syringes. (Need I add that illicit use of drugs and alcohol is irresponsible and highly dangerous, whether or not sex is involved?)

5. Beware, especially, of male homosexual union. The warnings above apply to heterosexuals and homosexuals, but especially to homosexual males, who are at greater risk because of the secrecy and daring that a disapproving society forces on them. Homosexuals seek like-attracted companions and sometimes find them in places where they---especially younger homosexuals---are vulnerable to **promiscuous predators**. (A reason to encourage a tolerant society in which homosexual adolescents can establish safe and steady romantic bonds without secrecy and without being condemned.) Among male homosexual predators are some aggressively masculine adults and adolescents who deny their homosexuality, not only to others but also to themselves. They prey on vulnerable boys in the name of "variety," and if they are infected with HIV and do not wear condoms during sexual activity, they will spread the infection not only to the boys they seduce or rape but also to their own wives and girl friends. This behavior pattern, currently called "the down low," is responsible for an alarming spread of AIDS among African-American adolescent and adult males and thus their girl friends and wives.

Sexual gratification between homosexual males is usually by mutual masturbation, oral sex, and anal intercourse. Any of these activities can induce HIV if a partner is infected and neither wears a condom, but anal intercourse is by far the riskiest. An infected partner who fails to wear a condom is certain to induce HIV when penetrating the anus of an uninfected partner. The reverse is also true: if an uninfected male penetrates, without condom, the anus of an infected partner.

Adolescents, especially boys, tend to think they are invincible, and they easily fall prey to people who entice them to experiment sexually without precautions such as condom use. The result has been, and is, an alarming increase of HIV infection among teenagers. This is a tragedy because AIDS is fatal, no matter how long it can be contained by expensive medication. (See Harvey Fierstein's article mentioned in the Bibliography.)

6. This, especially, to be discussed with parents: Whether you are male or female, heterosexual or homosexual, get accustomed to the practice of having a package of fresh condoms available, if not for your own use, then for giving to others. "Unprotected" sexual coupling (engaging in sexual activity without condoms) is adding risk to risk, and you owe it to yourself and to your friends to be so protected and protective. I write this hoping and assuming nonetheless you will uphold the values of respect, trust, and responsibility---avoiding promiscuity---that I have stressed throughout this book.

7. If you are injured (cuts and other abrasions), avoid contact of such injuries with the blood, semen, saliva, or vaginal secretions of anyone suspected or known to have HIV.

8. If you are scheduled for surgery that may require blood or plasma transfusion, ask your physician about the possibility of your donating, ahead of time, your own blood for transfusion. Blood donors are carefully screened for infections, and donated blood is carefully tested for antibodies that indicate infection, but there remains a remote possibility of negative-testing blood drawn from a person infected with HIV even months earlier. (Of course, that person would be disgracefully irresponsible in donating blood!)

Now, what not to fear.

1. People who have HIV, whether or not it has developed into full-blown AIDS, are not infectious unless one comes in contact with their bodily fluids---blood, semen, vaginal secretions, and, to a lesser extent, breast milk---in their liquid state. Even so, these fluids would have to enter through abrasions or through oral, vaginal, or anal orifices. (Sweat and tears, by the way, are not sources!) Of course, people with HIV are responsible for telling their employers, their families, their close friends, and any group with which they are in frequent and possibly close contact. No matter how embarrassing, and no matter how the HIV was acquired, this is an ethical and moral requirement. Magic Johnson, the basketball star, has been a good role model in this respect. So was Arthur Ashe, the great tennis star, who acquired HIV from infected blood transfusion.

2. No matter whether the HIV-infected person is an employee, employer, student, teacher, friend, acquaintance, family member, or any other category, there is no harm in sitting next to that person, shaking hands, conversing, doing business, eating dinner, carrying on in all the normal day-to-day activities. Even such an intimacy as a kiss on the cheek is harmless. Employment of HIV-infected people in kitchens and at table waiting is also harmless. So also is use of toilet facilities after use by an HIV-infected person. One should not increase the doomsday burden of an HIV-infected person by shunning him or her, especially out of ignorance. We have a responsibility to accept such infected people as fellow human beings.

3. People donating blood for transfusions are in no danger of HIV infection, but of course they should not volunteer to donate blood if their own sexual activity is at all promiscuous or risky.

Final Thoughts on STDs

The subject of sexually transmitted diseases is not what one discusses happily, but it is, as you must surely see, vital to your lifelong health, your reputation, and your self-esteem. When you have fallen in love with the person you desire as a lifetime partner, you won't want to be in the situation of having to say, in this connection, "There's something I ought to tell you . . . "

Now, let's move from these heavy consequences to the conclusion of this book and to the happy consequences of responsible love and sex.

Conclusion

Getting back to the beginning, and to the purposes of this book. You are reading this book, partly out of curiosity, possibly because your parents or some other caring adult gave it to you, and---most important---because you are *here*: lovingly conceived and brought into this world to live happily, to make this world a better place for your being here, and to lovingly, responsibly, and hopefully fulfill the biological imperatives of sexual pleasure and reproduction.

I have tried to show you that sexual behavior, like all other behavior, has its consequences---wonderful and good when responsible, dangerous for you and harmful to others when irresponsible. There are a few places where you might accuse me of being preachy. I won't apologize for that. I avoided, however, getting into judgments on good and evil. Such judgments are better left to your parents and religious counselors and to you in the culture in which you are brought up. Instead, I've tried to be realistic about situations that confront you in this increasingly tempting and complicated society we live in. And I've tried to compliment you with your ability to make mature judgments for yourself *so that you can avoid now the mistakes for which you would later curse yourself.* Moreover, I have many times expressed the hope that you and your parents can and will discuss any and all of the ideas that I have provoked. You and your parents may find such discussion difficult and embarrassing at first, but eventually helpful and rewarding.

Goodbye, and best wishes for a happy and loving life!

Bibliography

Entries preceded by an asterisk (*) are especially valuable for further study.

*Araton, H. "Sports of the Times: The Wall of Silence Is Crumbling in Baseball." *The New York Times.* New York, NY: February 29, 2004.

*Arledge, E. and Cort, J. *Cracking the Code of Life.* NOVA, WGBH/Boston Video. South Burlington, VT: 2001.

*Beers, M. H. and Berkow, R., eds. *The Merck Manual of Diagnosis and Therapy, 17th Edition.* Merck & Co., Inc. New York, NY: 1999.

Bellafante, G. "Two Fathers, With One Happy to Stay at Home." *The New York Times.* New York, NY: January 12, 2004.

Bernstein, F. A. "On Campus, Rethinking Biology 101." *The New York Times.* New York, NY: March 7, 2004.

Betrayed: Update on Sexual Misconduct in Schools. Hendrie, C., "Part One: States Target Sexual Abuse by Educators," April 30. Hendrie, C., "Part Two: Family Heals After Teacher-Student Relationship," May 7. *Education Week.* Bethesda, MD: 2003.

*Bowman, D. H. "Abstinence-Only Debate Heating Up." *Education Week*. Bethesda, MD: February 11, 2004.

*Bowman, D. H. "Report Says Schools Often Ignore Harassment of Gay Students." *Education Week*. Bethesda, MD: June 6, 2001.

Bowman, D. and Gehring, J. "Policymakers Tackling Teenage Steroid Abuse." *Education Week*. Bethesda, MD: April 21, 2004.

*Brody, J. E. "Abstinence-Only: Does It Work?" *The New York Times*. New York, NY: June 1, 2004.

*Brody, J. E. "Children, Media and Sex: A Big Book of Blank Paages." *The New York Times*. New York, NY: January 31, 2006.

*Brody, J. E. "Condoms Stay Faithful When Prevention Is the Goal." *The New York Times*. New York, NY: August 22, 2006.

*Brody, J. E. "Empowering Children to Thwart Abductors." *The New York Times*. New York, NY: January 28, 2003.

Brody, J. E. "Getting to Know a Virus, and When It Can Kill." *The New York Times*. New York, NY: October 18, 2005.

Brody, J. E. "Regular Pap Tests Remain a Crucial Detection Method." *The New York Times*. New York, NY: July 31, 2001.

Brody, J. E. "Yeast Infection: The Pitfalls of Self-Diagnosis." *The New York Times*. New York, NY: March 19, 2002.

*Brooks, D. "The Power of Marriage." *The New York Times*. New York, NY: November 22, 2003.

*Carey, W. B. *Understanding Your Child's Temperament,* revised edition. New York, NY: MACMILLAN, 2005.

Cloud, J. "AIDS at 20." *TIME*. New York, NY: June 11, 2001.

Consumers Union of United States, Inc. and B. Winikoff and S. Wymelenberg. *The Contraceptive Handbook.* Consumer Reports Books. Yonkers, NY: 1992.

*Cort, J. and Nilsson, L. *Life's Greatest Miracle.* NOVA, WGBH/ Boston, PBS Home Video, South Burlington, VT: 2001.

*Denizet-Lewis, B. "Double Lives on the Down Low." *The New York Times Magazine.* New York, NY: August 3, 2003.

Ebert, J., Loewy, A., et al. *Biology.* New York, NY: Holt Rinehart and Winston, 1973.

*Egan, T. "Body Conscious Boys Adopt Athletes' Taste for Steroids." *The New York Times.* New York, NY: November 22, 2002.

Eisenberg, M. E., et al. "Parents' Beliefs About Condoms and Oral Contraceptives: Are They Medically Accurate?" *Perspectives on Sexual and Reproductive Health, Volume 36, Number 2.* The Alan Guttmacher Institute. New York & Washington: March/April, 2004.

*Eisner, J. "Girls Left Wounded by a Hookup Culture." *The Philadelphia Inquirer.* Philadelphia, PA: June 6, 2004.

*Eisner, J. "Sex Education for Teens Needs a Dose of Reality." *The Philadelphia Inquirer.* Philadelphia, PA: March 7, 2004.

*Fierstein, H. "The Culture of Disease." *The New York Times.* New York, NY: July 31, 2003.

Fischer, K. W. and Lazerson, A. *Human Development, from Conception Through Adolescence.* New York, NY: W. H. Freeman and Company, 1984.

Fisher, W. and Hoffman, D. "Adolescence: A Risky Time. Why teenagers won't---or can't---take the threat of AIDS seriously." *Independent School.* National Association of Independent Schools. Washington, D.C.: Spring, 1992.

Florio, G. "Kids & Sex." *The Philadelphia Inquirer.* Philadelphia, PA: August 8, 1999.

Friend, R. "Listening to Silenced Voices. Strategies for undoing homophobia in schools." *Independent School.* National Association of Independent Schools. Washington, D.C.: Spring, 1992.

Galley, M. "New School Curriculum Seeks to Combat Anti-Gay Bias." *Education Week.* Bethesda, MD: November 3, 1999.

Gilbert, S. "Teaching Teenagers a Subject Many Know All Too Well." *The New York Times.* New York, NY: October 10, 2000.

*Ginsberg, T. "Cervical-Cancer Vaccine Cleared." *The Philadelphia Inquirer.* Philadelphia, PA: June 9, 2006.

Hacker, A. "Gays and Genes." *The New York Review of Books.* New York, NY: March 27, 2003.

Hall, S. S. "Bully in the Mirror." *The New York Times Magazine.* New York, NY: August 22, 1999.

*Haney, D. Q. "N.C. Finds a Puzzling Jump in HIV." *The Philadelphia Inquirer.* Philadelphia, PA: February 11, 2004.

Hendrie, C. "Experts Convene on Sexual Abuse by Teachers." *Education Week.* Bethesda, MD: April 9, 2003.

Hendrie, C. "No Easy Answers for Schools in Misconduct Inquiries." *Education Week.* Bethesda, MD: May 7, 2003.

Hepola, S. "Her Favorite Class: 'Sex' Education." *The New York Times.* New York, NY: June 22, 2003.

Hiltbrand, D. "Online, Out of Control." *The Philadelphia Inquirer.* Philadelphia, PA: November 2, 2003.

*Honawar, V. "Abstinence-Only Curricula Misleading, Report Says," *Education Week.* Bethesda, MD: December 8, 2004.

Hurst, M. "High School Students to Ask for Change in Sex Education." *Education Week.* Bethesda, MD: October 17, 2001.

Is Homosexuality Biologically Influenced? A Debate. LeVay, S. and Hamer, D. H., "Evidence for a Biological Influence in Male Homosexuality." Byne, W., "The Biological Evidence Challenged." *Scientific American.* New York, NY: May 1994.

Jacobs, A. "The Beast in the Bathhouse: Crystal Meth ['Ice'] Use by Gay Men Threatens to Reignite an Epidemic." *The New York Times.* New York, NY: January 12, 2004.

Johnson, E. W. *Love and Sex in Plain Language.* New York, NY: Bantam Books, Inc. 1974.

Kinsey, A. C., et al. *Sexual Behavior in the Human Female.* Philadelphia, PA: W. B.Saunders Company, 1953.

Kinsey, A. C., et al. *Sexual Behavior in the Human Male.* Philadelphia, PA: W. B.Saunders Company, 1948.

*Kirn, W. "Sex-Ed Night School." *The New York Times Magazine.* New York, NY: November 16, 2003.

*Klitzman, R. and Bayer, R. *Mortal Secrets: Truth and Lies in the Age of AIDS.* New York, NY: Columbia University Press, 2003.

*Kristof, N. D. "Gay at Birth?" *The New York Times.* New York, NY: October 25, 2003.

*Kristof, N. D. "No Time to Get Squeamish." *The New York Times.* New York, NY: May 9, 2003.

*Landry, D., Darroch, J., et al. "Factors Associated with the Content of Sex Education in U.S. Public Secondary Schools." *Perspectives on Sexual and Reproductive Health, Vol. 35, No. 6.* The Alan Guttmacher Institute. New York & Washington: November/December, 2003.

*Lerner, S. "Making New Efforts to Convince Youths They Are Not Invulnerable to H.I.V." *The New York Times*. New York, NY: August 5, 2003.

Lewin, Tamar. "1 in 5 Teenagers Has Sex Before 15, Study Shows." *The New York Times*. New York, NY: May 20, 2003.

Lewis, W. H., ed. *Gray's Anatomy of the Human Body, 20th edition*. New York, NY: Bartleby.com, 2000.

*Longman, J. "An Athlete's Dangerous Experiment." *The New York Times*. New York, NY: November 26, 2003.

Maeroff, G. I. "The 'Wedge Issues' of 2004: Why Educators Should Be Wary." *Education Week*. Bethesda, MD: January 7, 2004.

Manlove, J. and Franzetta, R. and K. "Patterns of Contraceptive Use Within Teenagers' First Sexual Relations." *Perspectives on Sexual and Reproductive Health, Vol. 35, No. 6*. The Alan Guttmacher Institute, New York & Washington: November/December, 2003.

Marano, H. E. "Sexual Issues Fan Parents' Fears." *The New York Times*. New York, NY: July 2, 1997.

Masters, W. H. and Johnson, V. E. *Human Sexual Response*. Boston, MA: Little, Brown, 1966.

*McLane, J. "Mind over Muscle: Confronting Steroid Temptation." *The Philadelphia Inquirer*. Philadelphia, PA: August 31, 2006.

*McCullough, M. "Just Saying 'No' to Pregnancy." *The Philadelphia Inquirer*. Philadelphia, PA: February 23, 2004.

McCullough, M. "Sex-Assault Treatment Guidelines Omit Pill." *The Philadelphia Inquirer*. Philadelphia, PA: December 31, 2004.

Meckler, L. "'Call to Action' on Sexual Values." *The Philadelphia Inquirer*. Philadelphia, PA: June 29, 2001.

Meckler, L. "Study: Condoms Don't Boost Teen Sex." *The Philadelphia Inquirer* Philadelphia, PA: May 29, 2003.

Navarro, M. "Spreading the Pope's Message of Sexuality and a Willing Spirit." *The New York Times.* New York, NY: June 7, 2004.

Neergaard, L. "More Virulent Strain of Chlamydia Rising Among Gay Men." *Associated Press* in *The Philadelphia Inquirer.* Philadelphia, PA: February 7, 2006.

Netter, F. H. *Atlas of Human Anatomy.* Summit, NJ: CIBA-GEIGY Corporation, 1998.

Planned Parenthood Federation of America, Inc., R. F. Moglia and J. Knowles, eds. *All About Sex: A Family Resource on Sex and Sexuality.* New York, NY: Three Rivers Press, 1997.

Reid, K. S. "School Pride." *Education Week.* Bethesda, MD: October 15, 2003.

"Research Shows Sperm Has Egg Locater." *The New York Times.* New York, NY: March 28, 2003.

*Samuels, C. "Abstinence Programs Lack Factual Reviews, GAO Study Concludes." *Education Week*. Bethesda, MD: November 29, 2006.

*Samuels, C. "'Choking Game' Yields Varying Responses from Educators." *Education Week.* Bethesda, MD: June 7, 2006.

*Satcher, D., Surgeon General of the United States. *The Call to Action to Promote Sexual Health and Responsible Sexual Behavior.* Department of Health and Human Services. Washington, D.C.: 2001. Currently unavailable to public

Schemo, D. J. "Mothers of Sex-Active Youths Often Think They're Virgins." *The New York Times.* New York, NY: September 5, 2002.

*Schemo, D. J. "Sex Education with Just One Lesson: No Sex." *The New York Times.* New York, NY: December 28, 2000.

*Schemo, D. J. "Surgeon General's Report Calls for Sex Education Beyond Abstinence Courses." *The New York Times*. New York, NY: June 29, 2001.

*Schemo, D. J. "Survey Finds Parents Favor More Detailed Sex Education." *The New York Times*. New York, NY: October 4, 2000.

Schemo, D. J. "What Teenagers Talk About When They Talk About Chastity." *The New York Times*. New York, NY: January 28, 2001.

Schiavo, C. "Alliance Is Looking Out for Rights of Gay Pupils." *The Philadelphia Inquirer*. Philadelphia, PA: June 14, 2003.

Schlosser, E. "Empire of the Obscene." *The New Yorker*. New York, NY: March 10, 2003.

Schrof, J. M. "Pumped Up." *U.S. News & World Report*. Washington, D.C.: June 1, 1992.

*Shorto, R. "Contra-Contraception." *The New York Times Magazine*. New York, NY: May 7, 2006.

Singer, S. and Hilgard, H. R. *The Biology of People*. San Francisco, CA: W. H. Freeman and Company, 1978.

*"Some Routine AIDS Screening Is Advised." *The New York Times*. New York, NY: April 18, 2003.

*"Steroids in Sports." Five articles in *The New York Times*. New York, NY: November 17-21, 1988.

Stolberg, S. G. "Grants Aid Abstinence-Only Initiative." *The New York Times*. New York, NY: February 28, 2002.

*Stolberg, S. G. "Men's Reproductive Health Care Gets New Emphasis." *The New York Times*. New York, NY: March 19, 2002.

Stolberg, S. G. "U.S. Awakes to Epidemic of Sexual Diseases." *The New York Times*. New York, NY: March 9, 1998.

Surendran, A. "Teens Take up Task of Sending Health Messages." *The Philadelphia Inquirer*. Philadelphia, PA: October 15, 2002.

Teenage Sexual and Reproductive Behavior in Developed Countries. "Country Report for the United States." Occasional Report No. 8. The Alan Guttmacher Institute. New York & Washington, Nov., 2001.

*Trotter, A. "U.S. Court Backs School's Decision to Bar Student's Anti-Gay T-Shirt." *Education Week*. Bethesda, MD: May 3, 2006.

A Trust Betrayed: Sexual Abuse by Teachers. Hendrie, C., "Part One: Sex with Students: When Employees Cross the Line," December 2. Hendrie, C., "Part Two: Cost Is High When Schools Ignore Abuse," December 9. Hendrie, C., "Part Three: 'Zero Tolerance' of Sex Abuse Proves Elusive," December 16. *Education Week*. Bethesda, MD: 1998.

Tuller, D. "Experts Voice New Alarm on Herpes." *The New York Times*. New York, NY: May 8, 2001.

Tuller, D. "New H.I.V. Test Offers Quicker Results, but the Same Anguish." *The New York Times*. New York, NY: June 1, 2004.

Tuller, D. "Some Urge Type of Pap Test to Find Cancer in Gay Men." *The New York Times*. New York, NY: February 18, 2003.

Wade, N. "Y Chromosome Depends on Itself to Survive." *The New York Times*. New York, NY: June 20, 2003.

*Wolf, N. *Promiscuities, the Secret Struggle for Womanhood*. New York, NY: A Fawcett Columbine Book, Ballentine Pub.Group, Div. of Random House, Inc., 1997.

Young Love, New Caution. Bernstein, N. "Behind Fall in Pregnancy, A New Teenage Culture of Restraint," March 7. "For a Promising but Poor Girl, a Struggle Over Sex and Goals," March 8. *The New York Times*. New York, NY: 2004.

*Zuger, A. "A Long Life? A Death Sentence? AIDS Still Offers No Easy Answers." *The New York Times*. New York, NY: June 6, 2006.

INDEX

115

About the Author

Edward Shakespeare, retired schoolteacher, received his B.A. degree in biology from Haverford College and his M.A. degree in embryology and histology from Cornell University. He began his teaching career in science, then worked as an editor with W. B. Saunders Company, medical publisher. A lover of literature and drama, as well as of science, he returned to teaching, first at The William Penn Charter School to chair the English department and then at Friends' Central School, where he also taught biology.

He is author and principal editor of several high-school textbooks, including *Understanding the Essay* and *Drama: From Print to Performance*; he has chaired the English committees of the National Association of Independent Schools and the Independent School Teachers Association of Greater Philadelphia; and he has served on the boards of Haverford College, Delaware Valley Friends School, and Green Tree School.

Once widowed, he has two sons by his first marriage, two stepchildren by his second marriage, and three stepgrandchildren.

Mr. Shakespeare has taught sex education as a part of biology curricula, including a brief collaboration with Dr. Alan Guttmacher (founder of the Alan Guttmacher Institute) at the Park School in Baltimore in 1951. Mr. Shakespeare began work on *Sex and Consequences* in 1980 but later put it aside until 2000. It is the result of years of observation of casual behavior and conversations among young and older teenagers in classrooms, homerooms, school social events, and carpools. Concerned now by increasing license in the various media and at school events and social settings, he believes that a fully informed bioethical approach to sex education is today a necessity.

www.ingramcontent.com/pod-product-compliance
Lightning Source LLC
Chambersburg PA
CBHW020252290526
45784CB00003B/1218